T0121184

THE

ABORTION RESOURCE HANDBOOK

K KAUFMANN

THE

ABORTION RESOURCE HANDBOOK

A FIRESIDE BOOK

Published by Simon & Schuster

This publication contains the opinions and ideas of its author. It is intended to provide helpful and informative material on the subject matter covered. It is sold with the understanding that the author and publisher are not engaged in rendering medical, legal, or other professional services in the book. If the reader requires personal, medical, or health assistance or advice, a competent professional should be consulted.

The author and publisher specifically disclaim any responsibility for any liability, loss, or risk, personal or otherwise, which is incurred as a consequence, directly or indirectly, of the use and application of any of the contents of this book.

FIRESIDE

Rockefeller Center

1230 Avenue of the Americas

New York, NY 10020

Copyright © 1997 by K Kaufmann

All rights reserved, including the right of reproduction
in whole or in part in any form.

FIRESIDE and colophon are registered trademarks of Simon & Schuster Inc.

Manufactured in the United States of America

1 3 5 7 9 10 8 6 4 2

Library of Congress Cataloging-in-Publication Data

Kaufmann, K
The abortion resource handbook / K Kaufmann.
p.   cm.
Includes bibliographical references and index.
1. Abortion—United States.   2. Abortion—Law and legislation—
United States.   3. Abortion services—United States.   4. Pregnancy,
Unwanted—United States.   I. Title.
HQ767.5.U5K38   1997
363.46'0973—dc21   97-10262
CIP

ISBN 0-684-83076-0

To the providers—the doctors, nurses, clinic administrators, counselors, and staff—who have worked tirelessly, with unfailing courage, and all too little recognition, to ensure that abortion remains safe, legal, affordable, and, to the greatest extent possible, a positive experience for all women

ACKNOWLEDGMENTS

From beginning to end, *The Abortion Resource Handbook* has been a collaborative effort, and I have been blessed, humbled, and inspired throughout by the generous support and encouragement I have received from everyone involved.

First, last, and always, this book would not have been possible without the many generous women who believed in the project and provided early support and funding through the unofficial "Prochoice Women's Committee." I cannot thank them enough for taking a chance on an idea and an unknown writer. I am also grateful to Susan Petro, Linda Jue at Media Alliance, and Joan Pinkvoss of Aunt Lute Press for essential legal advice and technical support during the initial stages of research and writing. The National Abortion Federation and its many members have also been unstinting in their support of the book, and I am particularly indebted to Gina Shaw, whose good name facilitated numerous contacts and interviews with abortion providers across the country.

The doctors, nurses, clinic administrators, and counselors I have spoken with over the past few years are, simply, beyond praise. There is not room to acknowledge everyone who responded so generously to my requests for interviews and information; however, I would like to thank the following individuals who answered questions and reviewed chapters: Anne Baker, Toni Bond, Jane Bovard, Barbara Calfee, Renee Chelian, Diane Derzis, Susan Dudley, Dr. Jerry Edwards, Dr. Bruce Ferguson, Kelly Groux, Diane Hale, Dr. Mildred Hansen, Stacey Haugland, Dr. Warren Hern, Peg Hill-Callahan, Dr. Herbert Jones, Jane Lee, Alice Malin, Gail McMahon, Beth Petzelt, Amy Pierpont, Dr. Suzanne Poppema, the Reverend Velvet Rieth, Robin Rothrock, Dr. Eric Schaff, Michelle Schlarmann, Joan Schrammeck, Leslie Sebastian, Lauren Shelton, Lauren

Simonds, Tammy Sobieski-Joy, Dale Steinberg, Sue Steketee, Eileen Tamsky, Deni Thurman-Eyer, Dr. George Tiller, Dena Vogler, Dona Wells, Tina Welsh, and Dr. Glenn Weyhrich.

Special thanks also to Barbara Faye Waxman for her input on access issues affecting women with disabilities; lawyers Amelia Adams, John Cowles, Julie Field, Al Gerhardstein, Nancy McMillen, Rachael Pirner, Jamie Sabino, and Jane Tucker for information on the judicial bypass process; Marlene Fried, Fran Chalin, Marnie Wells, Kathy Ward, and other members of the National Network of Abortion Funds for help with the funding chapter; Brenda Cummings for her wealth of information on geographic access issues; veteran clinic defenders Joan Clark and Laura Weide for their help and feedback on the clinic harassment chapter; Jean Stewart Berg of the Religious Coalition for Reproductive Choice for her insights on the spiritual and emotional issues surrounding women's abortion decisions; Jule Hallerdin of Johns Hopkins School of Nursing for her careful review of Chapter 8: Taking Care of Yourself; Sandra Waldman at the Population Council for keeping me up to date on mifepristone; Molly A. Minnick of *A Heartbreaking Choice* for providing essential materials on the sensitive issue of late abortion; Ann Daniels of the California Abortion and Reproductive Rights Action League for help with the state-by-state list; Sarah Baker, editor extraordinaire; and the on-line pro-choice community—especially Victoria Tepe, Adam Guasch-Melendez, Ann Rose, and other members of "Jane"—for quick answers to picky questions. The Center for Reproductive Law and Policy, the Feminist Majority Foundation, and the Alan Guttmacher Institute also responded enthusiastically to my many and repeated requests for publications and information.

I have been extremely fortunate to find a publisher like Simon & Schuster who understood the importance of this book and has remained entirely committed to the project and its success, even in the midst of threatened boycotts by antichoice groups. I am also grateful to my agent, Felicia Eth, for her patience, careful readings, and insightful feedback.

Encouragement and support throughout the long months of research and writing have come from my parents, Karl and Elaine Kaufmann, as well as members of my San Francisco family: Sheppard Kominars, Marv Appelbaum, Mary Connor, Karen Schiller, Darlene Pagano, Annette Weathers, Erin Blackwell, Margery Kreitman, Judith Knoop, MaryAnn Greenwood, and Susan Stone. I also wish to acknowledge the support of Cindy Arnold and, for transcription services and friendship above and beyond the call of duty, Michaele Reppas. My partner, Nora McLoughlin, provided research assistance, helpful suggestions, backrubs, love, laughter, and the incomparable gift of herself.

Finally, I wish to thank the brave and remarkable women who shared their abortion stories with me. At a time when women's access to abortion is increasingly at risk, their decision to take action and speak out will, I hope, inspire others to do the same.

CONTENTS

THE

ABORTION RESOURCE HANDBOOK

INTRODUCTION

If you are holding this book, you may be pregnant and may not want to be. You may have already decided to have an abortion, or you may still be considering your options. You may also feel worried, confused, frustrated, angry, or just plain scared.

That's understandable. While abortion has been legal in the United States since 1973, in the past 20 years women's ability to terminate unplanned pregnancies has been steadily undermined. Since the passage of the Hyde Amendment in 1976, Medicaid funding for abortion has been cut or severely restricted in 33 states, putting the procedure out of reach for thousands of low-income women. Informed consent and parental notification and consent laws were ruled constitutional in 1992, and state-mandated lectures, waiting periods, and laws that require minors to tell their parents or go to court for a special hearing are now in force in 29 states.

Antichoice violence and lack of training for physicians have also resulted in fewer providers—clinics and private doctors who perform abortions. According to the Alan Guttmacher Institute, the number of abortion providers in the United States has dropped 18 percent since 1982. Across the country, 84 percent of counties have no provider, and only 13 percent of all medical residency programs make learning the procedure mandatory. Today, 1 woman in 10 drives over 50 miles to get to the nearest provider, and 1 in 20 drives over 100 miles. In 1992, the American Civil Liberties Union's Reproductive Freedom Project found that 20 percent of all women seeking an abortion in the United States were unable to get one, either because they couldn't find or get to a provider or because they didn't have the money.

As if practical problems were not enough, the difficulties of getting an abortion are often intensified by the social stigma and need for secrecy that continue to surround the procedure. Although abortion is a common experience—in the United States, an estimated 1.3 million women terminate pregnancies every year—if you are feeling alone and isolated, it can be like reinventing the wheel.

The Abortion Resource Handbook was conceived and written to provide women with the support and clear, practical information they need to get an abortion regardless of their personal situation or the restrictive nature of the laws, lack of clinics, or level of antichoice violence in their state. My focus throughout the book is on demystifying current obstacles by letting women know what to expect and how to minimize any problems they encounter. Individual chapters have been reviewed by doctors, clinic administrators, and other prochoice professionals to ensure their accuracy. I have also tried to make the book as user-friendly as possible, so women can quickly find and read the chapters and sections they need and skip the ones that may not apply to their situation. Each chapter begins with an introductory heading identifying the issue and information it covers—such as informed consent laws or clinic harassment—and ends with an "At a Glance" checklist that can be skimmed for basic facts and quick tips.

Chapters 1 through 6 cover logistics: how to choose a clinic, deal with informed consent and parental notification and consent laws, and find help if you think you can't afford an abortion or have to travel to a clinic in another city or state. Chapter 7 contains information on clinic harassment, and Chapter 8 looks at the emotional and physical experience of unplanned pregnancy. Chapters 9 and 10 provide basic medical information on abortion, including the procedures used for first- and second-trimester abortions, what will be happening during your appointment, and the drugs that can be used for emergency contraception and early abortion. Chapter 11 is intended only for women who are having a late abortion because of a fetal anomaly or other life-threatening medical condition. The appendixes include a state-by-state list of laws and prochoice organizations; a resource and bibliography section; and sample parental notification, judicial bypass, and medical informed consent forms.

Abortion laws in the United States are currently in a state of flux and are likely to remain that way for years to come. The impact of the antichoice movement has so shifted the center of debate that many supposedly "prochoice" politicians now support informed consent and parental involvement laws and bans on certain late-abortion procedures. Even the long-awaited introduction of the "French abortion pill," RU-486 (mifepristone), cannot ensure that safe, legal, and affordable abortion will be equally available to all women. And nothing seems likely to stop the growth of virulent antichoice activism and violence. Under the circumstances, while every effort has been made to ensure the accuracy of this book, you should check with your provider or local prochoice organization for the most up-to-date information on laws and other conditions affecting the availability of abortion in your state.

If there is any irony or hope to be drawn from the current situation, it lies in the extraordinary resourcefulness and determination individual women have used to overcome any obstacles in their way. Yes, getting an abortion can be hard and intimidating. It may take more time and money, and it will almost certainly be more stressful, but *you can do it*. Abortion up to the 24th or 25th week of pregnancy is legal in all 50 states and U.S. territories and possessions, and help is available from clinics and a growing number of prochoice organizations and resources.

In writing this book, I have spoken with many women who have recently had abortions, and their stories have been both infuriating and inspiring. While using their voices, I have changed names and personal details to protect their anonymity.

No woman should have to risk her health, safety, or emotional well-being to get an abortion. *The Abortion Resource Handbook* will provide women with a more positive and empowering frame of reference within which to make their decisions and exercise their inalienable right to reproductive choice.

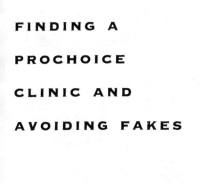

FINDING A PROCHOICE CLINIC AND AVOIDING FAKES

Read this chapter if you are pregnant, or think you might be, and want to find an abortion provider in your area—or if you just want to find a prochoice clinic where you can get a pregnancy test and talk with a counselor about your reproductive options.

If you have decided to have an abortion—or if you are pregnant and still unsure about your options—you will need to find a prochoice clinic. The clinic you choose is critical because it will determine the quality of care you receive before, during, and after the procedure. For many women, prochoice clinics provide a positive—and sometimes the only—source of support during a difficult time in their lives.

Unfortunately, for an increasing number of women, finding the appropriate clinic or doctor will involve more than just opening up the phone book and calling the local Planned Parenthood. Today, 84 percent of all counties in the United States have *no* abortion provider. This means that you may not have all the options you want when it comes to choosing a clinic. It does not mean, however, that you, or any other woman, should have to compromise on the basic quality of care you receive.

Medical treatment that is both competent and sensitive to your emotional needs is a right, not a privilege. Regardless of how old you are, where you come from, how much money you have, or the reasons you are seeking help, *you deserve good care.* This chapter contains information that will help you feel confident and comfortable about the clinic or doctor you select. The topics covered include:

- How to find the prochoice clinic or doctor nearest you
- What questions to ask the provider
- How to identify and avoid phony clinics run by antichoice organizations

WHAT IS A PROCHOICE CLINIC?

Prochoice clinics or medical practices are licensed medical facilities that are staffed by specially trained professionals, including doctors, nurses, and counselors, and equipped to provide a wide range of women's health care services. Most perform pelvic and breast examinations and offer family planning information, birth control, and prenatal care as well as pregnancy testing and abortions. They also diagnose and treat sexually transmitted diseases (STDs), vaginal infections, and other gynecological problems.

Equally important, counseling and other services at prochoice clinics are *nondirective and nonjudgmental.* Doctors, nurses, and counselors won't try to talk you into doing anything you don't want to do—either terminating a pregnancy or continuing it. They won't try to make you feel ashamed or guilty about being pregnant. Instead, they will give you information on your options, talk with you about your feelings, and encourage you to choose the course of action that is best for you.

In addition, at most prochoice clinics no woman will have an abortion until she has talked privately with a counselor, and the clinic is sure she is not being pressured or coerced to terminate or continue a pregnancy against her will. For example, a woman's partner may say he will leave her if she doesn't have an abortion, or a teenager's parents may threaten to throw her out of the house if she does. In most cases, if you tell a counselor you don't want to have an abortion, the clinic will postpone the procedure and provide you with additional counseling or referrals for prenatal care.

CALL NOW!

Some women find it hard to make that first call to a clinic. They may put it off for days or weeks, even if they only want to get a pregnancy test or speak with a counselor. Some women may delay calling because they have irregular periods and aren't sure if they're pregnant—or are afraid of finding out that they are. Others may worry that a partner, friend, or family member will find out that they are considering an abortion.

Misinformation is another reason for delay. Women who live in states with informed consent or parental notification and consent laws sometimes think that abortion is illegal—it's not—or are worried about being able to comply with the laws. Some women may have seen antichoice brochures that grossly misrepresent the dangers of abortion, stating, for example, that the procedure will make them sterile or increase their risk for breast cancer. Others may be afraid of having to go through picket lines of antichoice protesters. Or they may simply feel overwhelmed by the practical problems involved in getting an abortion, such as finding a ride to the clinic or the money to pay for the procedure.

While fear and delay are common, and understandable, *the sooner you call a clinic, the more time and options you will have.* Only about half of all clinics perform abortions in the second trimester—after the 12th or 13th week of pregnancy—and the procedure usually costs more and may require several appointments over a 2- to 3-day period (see **Second-Trimester Abortions,** page 9). If you need to go to a clinic in another city or state, travel expenses can add $100 or more to the cost of your abortion, and taking time off from work, arranging child care, or coming up with excuses for friends and family may also be more difficult and stressful. In addition, many providers only perform abortions a few days a week, and you may have to wait a week or longer for the first available appointment at a clinic in a small town or rural area.

In the end, many women find calling a clinic much easier and more reassuring than they expected. Many providers now have 800 numbers so that women can call for free, and any call or appointment you make will be strictly confidential. Counselors can answer your questions about the laws currently in force in your state, what to do if you're under 18 and don't want to tell your parents, or how to get past an antichoice picketer. In some cases, you may even be able to get a referral to a group who will help you pay for your abortion or give you a ride or a place to stay overnight. Here's how to find the clinic nearest you.

National Referral Lines

The quickest way to find a prochoice clinic in your area is to call the National Abortion Federation or Planned Parenthood referral lines.

- National Abortion Federation   800-772-9100 (United States)
       800-424-2280 (Canada)
- Planned Parenthood   800-230-7526

The **National Abortion Federation** (NAF) is a national organization of clinics and doctors dedicated to keeping abortion safe and accessible to all women. With over 300 clinics around the country, NAF-affiliated providers now perform about half of all abortions in the United States. Members also comply with the organization's code of professional standards, which includes a commitment to provide abortion services to women with disabilities and women with HIV/AIDS.

NAF's referral line is open Monday and Thursday, 9:30 A.M. to 1:30 P.M. and Wednesday and Friday, 9:30 A.M. to 5:30 P.M. eastern time. Callers are given the name and telephone number of the NAF member nearest them. Counselors on the line can also answer general questions about the abortion procedure and provide referrals to groups that help women pay for abortions (see **Chapter 5**). All calls are free and confidential, and you will not have to give the counselor your name or any other personal information.

The **Planned Parenthood** number connects callers to an electronic referral system. When you dial the number, a computerized system automatically switches your call to the Planned Parenthood clinic nearest you. The line is open 24 hours a day, 7 days a week; however, in most cases you should call during normal business hours in your area to make sure you speak directly to the clinic. If you call during nonbusiness hours, you may get a voice mail or answering machine and may have to leave a message.

While most Planned Parenthood clinics provide a full range of reproductive health services, some offices do not perform abortions. If you are switched to a clinic where abortion is not available, you will be referred to another Planned Parenthood office or prochoice provider in your area. Referral policies vary from office to office. In some cases, you may be required to go in for a pregnancy test and counseling before receiving a referral; in others, no appointment is required, and referrals are given directly over the phone.

The Yellow Pages

If you use your local Yellow Pages to find a clinic, be sure to look under **Abortion Providers** or **Abortion Services,** *not* Abortion Alternatives. Clinics under Abortion Alternatives are usually phony clinics run by antichoice organizations (see **Phony Clinics and How to Avoid Them,** page 13).

In most Yellow Pages, the Abortion Providers or Abortion Services heading includes a statement that identifies the clinics listed there as abortion providers. The statement will appear right under the heading and will read something like this:

> *Intended for businesses that provide abortion services or refer clients to businesses that do*

Going On-Line

Many prochoice organizations and some individual clinics now have home pages on the World Wide Web. At present, the top three Web sites for clinic referrals are the NAF and Planned Parenthood home pages and Abortion Clinics OnLine.

- NAF   http://www.prochoice.org/naf

- Planned Parenthood   http://www.ppfa.org/ppfa

- Abortion Clinics OnLine   http://www.gynpages.com

These sites include state-by-state clinic listings, links to individual clinic home pages, and links to information on abortion, birth control, and other women's health care issues. While quick, easy, and confidential, clinic listings on-line are somewhat limited at this time, and you may not be able to find a referral to a clinic near you at any of these sites. If that occurs, more detailed information on clinics in your area should be available from the NAF or Planned Parenthood referral lines.

WHAT QUESTIONS TO ASK

When you call a clinic for the first time, you will probably have questions about the facility and its abortion and counseling services. Asking questions at this point is important because it will help you evaluate the clinic and the quality of care you are likely to receive there.

If you feel scared or nervous about calling, write down your questions ahead of time, and don't worry about asking questions you think are dumb or too simple. Any clinic or private physician should be willing to answer any questions you have about the services they offer. In fact, many abortion providers say the sign of a really good clinic is how willing staff members are to answer women's questions fully and carefully over the phone.

"When I look at evaluating clinics, what's important to me is availability of information and how forthright they are," says Tammy Sobieski-Joy, director of a clinic in Florida. "I also listen to how the staff sounds on the phone. Do they sound professional? Do they sound like they really care about what you're saying? Are they just throwing information at you and saying good-bye, or do they really try to focus on your individual needs so you can make the decisions that are best for you?"

Of course, every woman will ask different questions, depending on her personal circumstances. Here are some of the questions you may want to ask:

+ *Do you perform abortions or refer to doctors who do?*

This the the first and most important question to ask, especially if you are unsure about whether you have called a phony clinic by mistake. A prochoice provider will give you a clear, straightfoward answer: "Yes, we do perform abortions," or "No, we don't do abortions, but we can refer you." If the person you speak with tries to avoid a direct answer or says something like "We can give you more information when you come in," the chances are strong that you are talking with a phony clinic.

+ *Are early and second-trimester abortions available? How late in the second trimester do you perform abortions?*

Until recently, most clinics would not perform an abortion until a woman was 6 or 7 weeks pregnant—measured from the first day of her last menstrual period. With current advances in reproductive health care and the introduction of the so-called abortion pills mifepristone, or RU-486, and methotrexate, some clinics now offer abortion as early as 3 weeks (see **Chapter 10**).

As noted, second-trimester abortions, that is, abortions after the 12th to 13th week, are available at about half of all clinics nationwide, but individual doctors and clinics vary in how late in the second trimester they will go. Some providers will only perform a second-trimester procedure up to the 16th or 18th week, while a few go as late as 24 or 25 weeks (see **Second-Trimester Abortions**, page 9).

+ *What type of abortion procedure will be done? What kind of anesthetics do you use?*

The standard procedure for abortions during the first trimester, or first 12 to 14 weeks of pregnancy, is vacuum aspiration. Most clinics prefer to use a local anesthetic, but intravenous (IV) sedation and general anesthetics are available at some facilities. Abortions during the second trimester are called D & Es, dilation and evacuation. The procedure requires two or more appointments and can be done either with a local or general anesthetic or with IV sedation (see **Chapter 9**).

♦ *Do you have a 24-hour emergency number?*

Although complications after an abortion are extremely rare—less than 1 percent of all cases—you should ask about the clinic's policy for treatment of complications and be sure a 24-hour emergency number is available. Most providers will have you return to the clinic for treatment except in real emergencies or if you live more than an hour or two from the clinic. In such cases, you may be told to go to a hospital emergency room.

Think twice before going to a provider that does not offer treatment for postabortion complications at the clinic. Going to an emergency room is expensive. Emergency room doctors are often unfamiliar with the treatment of postabortion complications and may perform unnecessary surgery. An emergency D & C—dilation and curettage, a procedure used to stop heavy bleeding—can cost anywhere from $500 to over $1,000, and in most cases you will have to pay all hospital fees yourself.

♦ *How much does it cost? What does the price include? When and how do I pay?*

Prices vary from clinic to clinic, but the average cost for a first-trimester abortion is now around $300 to $350. Private doctors usually charge more, about $400 and up, and costs will vary widely depending on the individual provider. In most cases, your abortion fee will include the procedure, pregnancy and other medical tests, counseling, a local anesthetic, treatment of postabortion complications at the clinic, and a follow-up examination 2 weeks later.

While price is a major concern for many women, keep in mind that when choosing a provider, cheaper is not always better, and be sure to ask about hidden costs. For example, does the fee cover all preabortion medical tests, including ultrasound, and postabortion medications, such as antibiotics to prevent infection, or Rho-gam if you are Rh-negative? Will IV sedation or a general anesthetic cost extra? (See **Chapter 9**.)

Also, find out what forms of payment or health insurance the clinic will accept. In general, clinics require payment in advance and do not accept personal checks. You will be expected to pay when you arrive for your appointment and will need cash, a credit card, or a bank check. If you live in a state that allows state funding for abortions and you qualify, you should find out what forms or documents you will need to bring.

♦ *Will I need to bring identification?*

Many clinics now require women to bring a current picture ID—a driver's license or passport—when they arrive for an appointment. This is done primarily for security reasons: to screen out antichoice protesters who may try to infiltrate the clinic by making an appointment under a false name. In states with parental consent laws, identification is also required to prove you are over 18. Most clinics do *not* require women to provide proof of citizenship or legal residency.

♦ *How soon can I make an appointment?*

Some clinics only perform abortions on certain days of the week or at certain times, and weekend or evening appointments are not always available. Where the clinic is the sole provider for a large geographic area, a woman may have to wait several days or weeks for an appointment.

Scheduling delays may also occur if you live in a state with informed consent or parental notification or consent laws. Many informed consent laws have 24-hour waiting periods, and two appointments at the clinic may be required (see **Chapter 2**). Some parental notification laws also have waiting periods—usually 24 or 48 hours—and if you decide not to tell your parents and go to court for a judicial bypass hearing, your abortion could be delayed several days, a week, or longer (see **Chapters 3 and 4**).

♦ *How long will I be at the clinic?*

Although a first-trimester abortion takes only about 5 to 10 minutes, you can expect to be at the clinic for 2 to 5 hours, on the average. Why do the appointments take so long? Part of the reason is that few clinics can afford to have a doctor on staff full-time. Abortions have to be scheduled when the doctor is available, and clinics do overbook.

In addition, the abortion procedure is only part of the care you will be receiving. Your appointment will include medical testing, counseling, and 20 minutes to an hour recovery time. Information on birth control and aftercare will be also discussed before you leave the clinic (see **Chapter 9**).

♦ *Can I bring a partner or friend? Can he or she stay with me during the procedure?*

Clinic policies on friends and partners vary widely. Many clinics allow partners, parents, or other support people to participate in preabortion counseling sessions if you want them to. Only a few allow friends and family in the procedure room during the abortion or in the recovery room afterward. You may also need someone to drive you to and from the clinic if you are having a second-trimester abortion or if any extra med-ication—valium, IV sedation, or a general anesthetic—is being used (see **Chapter 9**).

♦ *Do you provide child care? Can I bring my kids to the clinic?*

In the 1970s and 1980s, many clinics tried to provide child care but have since discontinued the service. Today, most clinics do not have child care on site, though a few may be able to refer you to local providers. Bringing children to the clinic is generally discouraged, and in some cases, a woman who arrives for an appointment with kids in tow will be asked to reschedule. If you have to bring your children to the clinic, also bring a partner or friend who can take care of the children during your appointment.

♦ *Do you have non-English-speaking staff? Can you provide translators for non-English-speaking women?*

The ability to provide translators for women who do not speak English varies according to the location of the clinic and its client demographics. For example, when a clinic has a large number of Latina clients, as many now do, it is likely they will have Spanish-speaking staff or will be able to arrange for a translator. In other instances, non-English-speaking women will need a friend or family member who can translate for them, both on the phone and during all appointments at the clinic. At some clinics, writ-ten materials on birth control and abortion may also be available in Span-ish or in a few Asian languages, such as Chinese, Vietnamese, or Tagalog.

SECOND-TRIMESTER ABORTIONS

As noted, while most providers perform abortions during the first trimester—up to the 12th or 13th week of pregnancy—only about half perform second-trimester procedures. The further along your pregnancy is, the harder it will be to find a provider and the more you can expect to pay.

The price for a second-trimester procedure varies greatly, depending on the individual provider and the length of your pregnancy. Prices range from $400 to over $2,500; in general, you can expect the cost to go up $50 to $100 for every 1 to 2 weeks of pregnancy. For example, a second-trimester abortion at 15 weeks will cost less than one at 18 weeks.

If you call a clinic that does not perform second-trimester abortions, the staff should be able to refer you to a provider that does. The NAF re-ferral line can also help you find a clinic or doctor in your geographic

---

WHAT TO LOOK FOR WHEN YOU GO TO THE CLINIC

When you go to a prochoice clinic, you should expect to see what you would see at any medical facility or doctor's office. The clinic should be clean and comfortable, the medical equipment should be modern and well-maintained, and the staff should be courteous and willing to answer any questions you have.

Renee Chelian, director of a clinic in Michigan, notes that even small details—like what kind of literature is in the waiting room—can tell women a lot about a provider. "When you walk in, there should be educational literature or brochures out in the waiting room, the furniture shouldn't be shabby, and there should be pictures on the wall," she says. "That tells you the clinic is interested in educating the patient and making her visit as comfortable and pleasant as possible."

Chelian and other providers also recommend that if possible, women visit a clinic at least once before the abortion. Going to a clinic for a pregnancy test or counseling is a good way to check out a provider beforehand, and many women find that having an extra appointment helps them feel more comfortable and confident about their abortion decision and the procedure itself.

---

area. For women in small towns or rural areas, the closest provider may be several hours away or in another state (see **Chapter 6**).

When you call a clinic, it is also important to know approximately how long you have been pregnant. Remember that providers vary in how late in a pregnancy they will perform a second-trimester abortion, and at most clinics, you will have a sonogram to confirm the length of your pregnancy. If you are uncertain about how long you have been pregnant, say so. *Don't lie.* If a clinic only performs abortions up to 16 weeks, and you are 19 weeks pregnant when you arrive for your appointment, you will probably be referred to another provider.

Keep in mind that a second-trimester abortion may take 2 to 3 days and two or more appointments may be required. If you are coming from another city or state, you may have to stay near the clinic overnight—at a hotel or with a friend—and you may need a friend to stay with you between appointments and drive you home after the procedure (see **Chapter 9**).

WOMEN WITH DISABILITIES

▼ Under the Americans with Disabilities Act (ADA), clinics are classified as public buildings and must be accessible to people with physical disabilities. Clinics should be located in buildings with ramps or elevators and wheelchair-accessible bathrooms. Waiting rooms, examination rooms, and other areas of the clinic should also be wheelchair-accessible.

While most clinics are wheelchair-accessible, and have been for a long time, services for women with physical disabilities or other special physical conditions may be lacking. Women with disabilities and very overweight women—300 pounds or more—are often told that they are high-risk clients and must be referred to a hospital. Most clinics do not have teletypewriter (TTY) phone equipment for deaf or hearing-impaired clients, and while some can provide American Sign Language (ASL) translation on request, many do not. Similarly, a few clinics have audiotapes for blind patients, but braille materials are generally not available.

Since the passage of the ADA, disability activists have been working with clinics to educate staff and improve access to reproductive health care, including abortion. In many cases, if you tell a clinic ahead of time the nature of your disability and the additional services you need, referral should not be necessary.

If you have a physical disability that makes it impossible for you to be examined in the traditional lithotomy (feet in the stirrups) position, alternative positions may be possible or the clinic may be able to get a specially equipped exam table. Disabled women should also be allowed to have an assistant or friend with them at all times during their appointment and abortion procedure. Women with hearing disabilities can have a signer in the room with them, and if you have a visual disability, you can bring an assistant or friend to describe what the doctor and clinic staff are doing during the abortion. Blind women can also ask to examine or feel all surgical instruments and the procedure room before the abortion, and music can be played during the procedure if you want.

A booklet entitled *Table Manners* is a good source of information on the services a clinic should be able to provide for women with disabilities. It is available from Planned Parenthood–Golden Gate, 815 Eddy Street, Suite 3000, San Francisco, CA 94109; 415-441-7858.

WOMEN WITH HIV/AIDS

▼ The ADA also makes it illegal for clinics to discriminate against or deny services to women with HIV or AIDS. Specifically, a clinic is not supposed to ask you if you are HIV-positive or refuse to terminate your pregnancy if you are. You do *not* have to tell clinic staff about your HIV status. If you do decide to tell, any information on your HIV status or current health should be kept confidential; however, the clinic may ask for copies of your current medical records, or you may have to get extra blood tests to make sure the procedure will be safe for you.

At present, most prochoice clinics perform abortions on HIV-positive women who have no AIDS-related symptoms or illnesses. If you have a very low T-cell count or other AIDS-related symptoms or illness, having an abortion could lead to further complications, and you may be referred to a hospital.

Keep in mind that most clinics now use universal precautions for all patients to prevent the spread of contagious diseases. Medical staff wear gloves and other protective clothing when performing examinations and surgical procedures, and medical equipment such as gloves, syringes, and pads are disposed of safely.

UNETHICAL PROVIDERS

As the number of doctors and clinics offering abortion services has declined, some supposedly prochoice providers have taken advantage of the situation by engaging in unethical practices such as overcharging women for medical tests or even performing unnecessary surgery. In many cases, these providers are located in inner-city areas and try to attract patients by advertising very low fees. The women most often targeted by these providers are those who have never been to a clinic before or have little experience in dealing with doctors or medical professionals in general, for example, teenagers and low-income or non-English-speaking women.

The scams used by unethical providers vary widely from city to city and clinic to clinic. In some cases, unethical providers simply offer very low-cost abortions and then add on lots of "extras," such as the medical tests and follow-up exams most clinics include in their basic fees. In others, providers deliberately give women inaccurate information on how long they have been pregnant so they can charge higher fees for an abortion.

For example, a woman who believes she is 10 weeks pregnant could be told that she is 14 weeks and needs to have a second-trimester procedure for an additional $150. Or the provider tells the woman that she is in the second trimester, refers her to another clinic, and then charges her a high fee—$100 or more—for an office visit and ultrasound. Women have also been offered menstrual extraction—a first-trimester abortion procedure using a handheld vacuum pump—even if they are not pregnant or have not had a pregnancy test.

To avoid unethical doctors or clinics, try to get complete information on a provider's fees and services before you make an appointment (see **What Questions to Ask,** page 5). If you think a provider may be engaging in unethical practices, call the NAF referral line or a local prochoice organization (see **Appendix 1**) and ask if they have ever received a complaint about the doctor or clinic you are concerned about.

If you go to a clinic where you do not feel safe or comfortable for any reason, you do *not* have to stay, even if you have already paid for an abortion or other medical treatment. You can leave, and demand your money back, at any time during your appointment. If you have had any medical tests, such as a pregnancy test or ultrasound, a small office fee may be deducted; $30 to $50 is reasonable. In other circumstances, and especially if you have not seen a doctor or counselor, your fee should be returned in full.

PHONY CLINICS AND HOW TO AVOID THEM

Phony clinics are facilities set up and run by antichoice organizations for the sole purpose of actively obstructing women's access to abortion. They do this primarily by giving women misleading or inaccurate information about pregnancy and abortion and by trying to make women feel scared, guilty, or ashamed about terminating an unplanned pregnancy. Advertising free pregnancy tests and confidential counseling, phony clinics often try to present themselves as a positive, caring alternative to prochoice facilities. In fact, these "clinics" and their antichoice tactics pose a real threat to women's health and emotional well-being.

To begin with, most phony clinics are *not* licensed medical facilities; it is illegal for them to perform medical procedures, such as pregnancy tests, or provide other health care services. In most cases, these facilities use the same kind of over-the-counter pregnancy test kits you can buy at a drugstore or supermarket. Women who have gone to phony clinics report that in some instances counselors have simply handed them a kit, told them to perform the test themselves, and then "interpreted" the results for them.

Over-the-counter tests are *not* medically reliable, so even if you use one at a phony clinic and get a positive result, you will still need to be retested when you go to a prochoice clinic or doctor. A valid pregnancy test is especially important for women who need written confirmation of their pregnancies to apply for state or federal funding for their abortions or other pregnancy-related medical or social services. *Tests performed at phony clinics are not considered valid by government or private social service agencies.*

In addition, the so-called counseling offered at phony clinics is *not* nonjudgmental and nondirective. In most cases, the people working at these facilities are *not* qualified medical personnel, such as doctors, nurses, and counselors who have received special training in women's health care. They are nonprofessionals who have been trained by anti-choice organizations to promote the political and religious beliefs advanced by these groups. Women who go to phony clinics are typically given inaccurate information, shown upsetting pictures and videos of dead fetuses, and subjected to other forms of emotional and physical harassment that can leave them feeling vulnerable, upset, and angry.

Recent investigations by prochoice groups have also revealed that some phony clinics are part of shady adoption rings. At these so-called crisis pregnancy centers, women who decide to continue their pregnancies are pressured, and at times physically coerced, into giving up their babies for adoption, most often to fundamentalist Christian families.

TESTS, LIES, AND VIDEOTAPE: JULIE'S STORY

Julie's story is typical of the kinds of lies and harassment women encounter when they go to phony clinics. A young woman in her early twenties, Julie was living in a small, isolated town in the Midwest when she got pregnant. Raised in a "liberal, prochoice household," she recalls that

---

WARNING: EVEN IF IT'S LICENSED, IT MAY STILL BE ANTICHOICE.

During the late 1980s and early 1990s, prochoice organizations repeatedly sued antichoice clinics for advertising themselves as licensed clinics when they were not. Now, antichoice organizations are setting up and advertising phony clinics that are medically licensed. This means the clinic can legally perform certain medical tests and procedures and may have a doctor or licensed counselor on staff. Evidence suggests that counseling at these facilities remains biased, however. Any woman who goes to an antichoice clinic, even a licensed one, can expect to receive inaccurate and misleading information about her pregnancy and her reproductive options, including abortion.

"I knew what my options were. I just wasn't sure which one was right for me."

With the nearest big city, and abortion provider, 3 hours away, Julie tried to find a nearby family planning clinic where she could get more information and counseling. She reports:

> I found this place in the Yellow Pages under the Abortion Information heading. It was called the Women's Pregnancy Center and was about twenty miles from where I lived. I called and said I had some questions and I wanted some information, and they said, come on in and bring your boyfriend with you. We went in, and the first thing they did was take a urine test. I knew just about exactly when I got pregnant—I was about two weeks at that point, but they told me I was almost two months. Then they said they had some tapes to show us. They put us in this little room and for a half an hour showed us tapes of abortion procedures. It was very graphic and antichoice—fetuses in garbage cans and everything short of you're going to hell if you have an abortion. I was very upset with the people there and told them that if they were a prolife outfit, they should present themselves as such and not as an unbiased information center.

Julie and her boyfriend left the clinic immediately, but the matter didn't end there:

> For the next three months, I got a postcard from them every other week. They would say things like, "We're praying for you and hope you make the right decision." I called them after I got the first card and said I would appreciate it if you would take me off your mailing list, but they didn't. It was unnerving, and I felt pretty angry about it.

With the support of her boyfriend, Julie decided to terminate her pregnancy. The clinic she chose is the sole provider for a large geographic area, so she had to wait over a month to get an appointment, by which time she was pretty close to the end of the first trimester.

Julie adds that the experience of the unwanted pregnancy and abortion brought her and her boyfriend much closer together. They are now married and recently had their first child.

HOW TO RECOGNIZE A PHONY CLINIC

Despite their very real differences, at first glance it may be hard to tell a phony clinic from a prochoice provider, says Leslie Sebastian, an administrator at a California clinic that has been in the forefront of efforts to expose the ways antichoice facilities trick and mislead women. "Women shouldn't blame themselves too much if they get duped into going to a phony clinic," she says. "These people are going out of their way to trick them."

If you're not sure whether a clinic is phony, call the NAF referral line or your state prochoice organization and ask if they know anything about the facility (see **Appendix 1**). Here are some of the telltale signs that will help you spot—and avoid—a phony clinic.

In Yellow Page Listings or Other Advertisements

Yellow Pages listings for phony clinics will appear under the Abortion Alternatives heading. In most cases, this heading will be followed by a statement that says the businesses listed here do *not* perform abortions. It will read something like this:

> *Intended for businesses that primarily provide assistance, counseling, and information on alternatives to abortion*

Display ads for phony clinics may be harder to identify. In most Yellow Pages, ads for prochoice and phony clinics often look similar and may even appear right next to each other, so you should read the ads carefully before you call. Here's what you'll probably see in ads for phony clinics:

+ A vague-sounding name, often with the word **pregnancy** in it; for example, Crisis Pregnancy Center, Pregnancy Help Center, or Problem Pregnancy Counseling

+ Offers of **"free pregnancy tests,"** often with immediate results, and **"walk-in appointments"**

+ Other misleading descriptions of available services, such as **"options counseling"** or **"postabortion counseling"**

Yellow Page directories are not the only places phony clinics advertise. Misleading ads may also appear in newspapers and magazines, and phony clinics often distribute flyers and brochures in their area. Remember also that just because a clinic is medically licensed does *not* mean it is prochoice, and a phony clinic may advertise itself as licensed even if it isn't.

On the Phone

Another easy way to identify a phony clinic is by how staff members respond to requests for information over the phone. Answers to even the most basic questions will be evasive and misleading, and callers will be encouraged to "come into the clinic for an appointment." For example, if you ask how much the clinic charges for an abortion, a staffer at a phony clinic might answer, "We can't give that information over the phone. Why don't you come in for an appointment, and we'll talk about it then."

Location

Phony clinics may be located on the same street or even in the same building as prochoice clinics, and their employees often try to intercept women arriving for appointments at the prochoice facility. In Dallas, Texas, women going to the prochoice Routh Street Clinic are sometimes approached by staffers from the White Rose Women's Center, a phony clinic with offices in the same building. Clad in white lab coats to look like medical personnel, the antichoice employees go up to women in the parking lot and say, "Hi! Are you going to the clinic? Come with me; I'm going up." In some cases, women have ended up in the phony clinic for several hours before realizing that the friendly person in a lab coat had deliberately misled them.

Note: If a clinic is regularly picketed by antichoice groups, women arriving for appointments may be met by client escorts—prochoice volunteers who will help them enter the building quickly and safely. Escorts often wear distinctive clothing, such as brightly colored T-shirts, vests, or armbands. If an antichoice picket is expected, your clinic will tell you whether, and where, to look for client escorts and how to identify them (see **Chapter 7**).

At the Clinic

Like their advertising and phone techniques, counseling and other practices at phony clinics are deliberately deceptive and misleading. First, phony clinics often ask women to provide personal information that has nothing to do with their pregnancy or medical history. For example, a medical history form might contain questions about your religious affiliation and whether you go to church, or a counselor might ask for your boyfriend's name, whether you're planning to get married, and what you or he think about abortion.

You should also check the small print on any forms you are asked to fill out and sign. Forms at phony clinics may include disclaimers stating that clinic personnel will break a woman's confidentiality if they believe she is going to harm her fetus. Women have reported instances where antichoice facilities have called their parents, or even local law enforcement or mental health agencies.

Finally, almost all phony clinics attempt to show women antichoice videos that contain inaccurate information and upsetting images of "aborted fetuses"—which are, in fact, stillborn babies. Typically, women are told they are going to see an "informational" video on abortion and are then taken to a viewing room. These rooms are often very small, and the women are not shown how to stop or turn off the tape player. In some cases, counselors have locked women and their partners in the room.

IF YOU GO TO A PHONY CLINIC BY MISTAKE

✔ If you discover you have gone to a phony clinic by mistake, *leave immediately.* People at the clinic may try to trick or intimidate you into staying or coming back for another appointment by saying that you can't leave until you have talked with a counselor or supervisor or that you should come back for another pregnancy test or more counseling. *None of this is true.*

Remember that you were tricked into going to the clinic in the first place. You do *not* have to be polite, listen to inaccurate or distorted information, or stay anywhere if you feel intimidated or uncomfortable.

Once you decide to leave, be firm and move quickly. Do *not* try to talk or argue with your counselor or other clinic personnel. Simply tell them you are leaving, you are not coming back, and the clinic is not to contact you again under any circumstances. If a phony clinic does try to call or threaten you in any way, call a prochoice clinic or group in your area and ask for help.

FINDING A CLINIC AND AVOIDING FAKES: AT A GLANCE

• When choosing a clinic, remember that *quality medical care is a right, not a privilege.* You deserve treatment that meets professional medical standards and is sensitive to your emotional needs.

• *Don't delay!* The sooner you call a prochoice clinic, the more time and options you will have.

* To find the prochoice clinic nearest you, call the **National Abortion Federation** at 800-772-9100 or **Planned Parenthood** at 800-230-7526. Clinic referrals are also available on-line at the NAF and Planned Parenthood Web sites and at **Abortion Clinics OnLine.**

* If you are looking for a clinic in the Yellow Pages, be sure you are looking under the **Abortion Provider** or **Abortion Services** heading, not **Abortion Alternatives,** where phony clinics are listed.

* Write down any questions you want to ask when you call the clinic, such as "Do you provide child care?" or "Can I bring a friend?" A good clinic will be glad to answer all your questions and will want to find out about your individual needs and concerns.

* Phony clinics run by antichoice organizations are generally *not* licensed medical facilities and do *not* provide medically accurate pregnancy tests or unbiased counseling. Women who go to phony clinics are usually given inaccurate or misleading information about abortion.

* To be sure you have not called a phony clinic by mistake, ask, "Do you perform abortions, or can you refer me to a provider who does?" The answer should always be yes.

* If you discover you have gone to a phony clinic by mistake, *leave immediately* and tell the people at the clinic that they are not to contact you under any circumstances.

* You can expect to pay $300 to $450 for a first-trimester abortion and $400 to over $2,500 for a second-trimester procedure. Abortion fees usually include all medical tests, counseling, treatment of postabortion complications, and a follow-up appointment.

* Women with disabilities or HIV/AIDS should *not* be referred to hospitals unless their condition requires extra medical backup. Most clinics use universal precautions to prevent the spread of infectious diseases and may be able to arrange special services with advance notice.

②

INFORMED

CONSENT

LAWS

AND

WAITING PERIODS

Read this chapter if you are going to a clinic in a state with an informed consent law. To find out about the law in each state, check the listings in **Appendix 1.**

Now in force in 11 states, so-called informed consent laws require women to receive state-mandated lectures and booklets on abortion and fetal development and then wait 24 hours before having an abortion. In many cases, the lecture must be given by a doctor or other medical professional, and women are required to make an extra appointment at the clinic just for the lecture, even if they are traveling from another city or state. The laws also state that women must be told they can see the booklets if they want to, but in most cases, they don't have to read or even look at them.

Informed consent measures have been supported by antichoice groups and legislators because, they say, the laws ensure that women considering abortion have full information on all their reproductive choices and take time to think carefully about their decisions. In fact, the laws cause many women unnecessary stress and delays, and the information in state-mandated lectures and booklets is often biased, inaccurate, and intended to make women feel scared or guilty about having an abortion. Waiting periods and extra appointments can also raise the cost of the procedure, especially for women who must take unpaid time off from work, drive long distances, arrange child care, or stay in a hotel overnight between appointments.

Informed consent laws seem even more unfair and frustrating because they are largely unnecessary. *Abortion is the only medical procedure to which informed consent laws currently apply. State-mandated materials and waiting periods are not required for any other kind of medical treat-*

ment or surgery. More to the point, women who go to prochoice clinics are already receiving medical informed consent counseling before their abortions. Providers report that the majority of women having abortions do think carefully about their decision before coming to the clinic. Women who receive state-mandated lectures and booklets often say the materials are "stupid," "condescending," or "boring" and have no impact on their decisions whatsoever.

If you are going to a clinic in a state with an informed consent law, your provider will be able to tell you what you will and won't have to do to comply with the law. Most providers are keenly aware of just how difficult it is for some women to come to a clinic twice and are doing everything they can to minimize the delays and other problems the laws can cause.

This chapter contains basic information on the informed consent laws currently in force in the United States. The material covered includes:

♦ What informed consent really means, and what prochoice clinics do, and have always done, to make sure women receive complete, unbiased information on all their reproductive choices

♦ The basic requirements of informed consent laws and what you may have to do to comply with them

♦ The information contained in state-mandated lectures and booklets, and the vital information they *don't* tell you

♦ What clinics are doing—and what you can do—to minimize the impact of informed consent laws

♦ What women and providers say about informed consent laws

WHAT IS INFORMED CONSENT?

Informed consent is the medical and legal term used to define a person's right to be given full information about any medical treatment she or he receives. In most cases, this information will include an accurate description of the treatment, its risks and benefits, and other options for care. Doctors and other medical professionals are also expected to be nondirective and nonjudgmental and to tailor any information they provide to the individual patient's needs and personal circumstances, such as age and education level. According to the American Medical Association, the purpose of informed consent is to create an opportunity for dialogue between patients and medical professionals and to allow patients to choose the treatment they feel is best for them.

Since the legalization of abortion in the early 1970s, prochoice clinics have pioneered the development of informed consent policies and practices to ensure that women facing unplanned pregnancies have full, unbiased information about all their reproductive options. Preabortion counseling sessions at most clinics are especially designed to make sure that women can ask questions about their pregnancies and the abortion procedure. Counselors also take time to talk with each woman privately to ensure that she feels comfortable with her decision and is not being pressured to continue or terminate a pregnancy if she doesn't want to (see **Chapter 9**).

Informed consent laws do not provide women with the accurate information contained in true medical informed consent counseling and are opposed by most prochoice doctors and clinics. Abortion is the only medical procedure to which these kinds of laws currently apply. Keep in mind also that state-prepared lectures and booklets are *not* replacing medical informed consent in any state, and whatever state-mandated materials you are given, you can still expect to receive full, unbiased counseling before your abortion.

THE LAWS

Informed consent laws usually have two basic requirements. First, the laws require that women receive a state-mandated lecture a certain period of time—usually 24 hours—before an abortion. The current exception to the rule is South Carolina, where the waiting period is only 1 hour.

The laws also state that women must be told that they can ask to see state-prepared materials on fetal development and the health and social services available to them if they decide to continue the pregnancy. The materials—usually booklets—are free of charge, and no woman has to look at them if she doesn't want to, except in Utah, where the law requires women to look at both a booklet and a video on fetal development. Failure to comply with an informed consent law is a criminal offense, and clinics and doctors who do not comply with the laws may be subject to fines or lose their licenses.

Note: Some informed consent laws contain emergency provisions that allow the state-mandated lecture and waiting period to be waived if continuing the pregnancy or delaying the abortion could put a woman's life at risk or cause permanent physical damage. A special form or letter from a doctor—usually, but not always, the one performing the abortion—is required, and not all doctors interpret the law, or what constitutes a life-endangering situation, in the same way. Doctors may grant a waiver if you are having an abortion because of a fetal anomaly, if the pregnancy is the result of rape or incest, or if you have a violent partner or parent and going to the clinic twice could put you at risk for physical abuse. Your clinic will be able to tell you whether the law in your state allows emergency waivers and what you will have to do to get one.

The following sections contain basic descriptions of the state-mandated lecture on abortion and the state-prepared booklets on fetal development and services for pregnant women. Of course, the exact wording of the lectures and descriptions of fetal development will vary, but in general, here's what you can expect.

The Lecture

Clinics in states with informed consent laws often give a special name to the state-mandated lecture to distinguish it from their regular preabortion counseling. A clinic in Utah calls the lecture the "state requirement." In Pennsylvania, it's the "information session." And Robin Rothrock, director of a clinic in Louisiana, says jokingly, "We call it the 'state harassment session.'" Most providers will also explain that they are required by law to give you the lecture, that it is not endorsed by the clinic, and that you will receive additional, unbiased counseling before your abortion.

In general, clinics try to keep the lectures as short and factual as possible. Most lectures last 5 to 15 minutes and include the name of the doctor who will perform the abortion, a description of the procedure to be used, information on the risks and benefits of abortion and childbirth, and how long you have been pregnant.

Informed consent laws in some states also require that certain misleading or partially true statements be included in the lecture. These kinds of antichoice statements are not wholly untrue, but they do not provide women with balanced or realistic information on all their reproductive options (see **What They Don't Tell You**, page 30). Depending on where you live, here are some of the antichoice statements you may hear.

‣ You may be eligible for financial support and free medical services from the state if you choose to carry your pregnancy to term.

- The father can be compelled to pay child support even if he has offered to pay for the abortion.

- You have the right to withdraw your consent to the abortion at any time before or during the procedure and may sue the doctor if she or he performs an abortion against your will.

- Having an abortion may increase your risk for breast cancer.

The Booklets

At some time during or at the end of the lecture, you will be told that you can ask to see the state-prepared booklets on fetal development and social services for women and children. In some states, the booklets are also available at family planning centers and public health clinics. *You do not have to read or even look at the booklets if you don't want to*—unless you live in Utah, where looking at the booklets is mandatory. If you do decide to look at the state-prepared booklets, here's what you can expect.

Fetal Development Booklets   State-prepared booklets on fetal development usually contain color photographs or, in a few cases, line drawings of the embryo and fetus at 2-week intervals from 4 to 40 weeks of gestation. The information accompanying the pictures includes the weight of the fetus, its length measured from the top of its head to the base of its spine—or "crown to rump," the term most doctors use—and details of its physical development. Some states also provide information on fetal viability—when and if the fetus can survive outside the womb—and descriptions of abortion procedures and different methods of birth control.

While seemingly accurate and professional-looking, fetal development booklets can be confusing and deceptive. Pictures of embryos and fetuses are often off-scale—either too large or too small—and the length of pregnancy may be measured from the probable date of conception, what is called gestational length, rather than from the first day of the last menstrual period, or LMP, the method most doctors use. Thus, a woman who has been told by her doctor that she is 8 weeks pregnant could look at a picture of an embryo labeled 8 weeks gestational—really, 10 weeks LMP—and think that her pregnancy is more advanced than it really is.

Line drawings in state-prepared booklets also overemphasize a fetus's human, babylike features, such as hair or plump arms and legs. Similarly, descriptions of fetal development focus on emotionally charged details of physical growth—for example, the development of fingernails or toenails—without providing accurate information on fetal viability (see **What They Don't Tell You,** page 30).

Information on abortion procedures and birth control may also be inaccurate and misleading. For example, some state-prepared booklets contain descriptions of a method of abortion called induction, an emotionally stressful procedure in which a woman is given drugs that cause her uterus to contract and the fetus to be "delivered." This was once the regular procedure for second-trimester abortions, but inductions are now performed only in a very small number of cases where a pregnancy is being terminated because of a fetal anomaly, and induction is the safest method to use (see **Chapter 11**).

Service Directories Service directories usually contain county-by-county listings of public, private, and nonprofit agencies that provide health and social services to pregnant women and their children. The organizations usually listed include state welfare offices, maternal and child health clinics, family planning centers, support and training programs for teen and single mothers, and so-called crisis pregnancy centers and adoption agencies. In most cases, only the address and phone number of the listed agencies are provided; information on the actual services offered and the organization's position on abortion may not be included.

Some of the listings in these books may, in fact, be helpful to women who are undecided about continuing or terminating a pregnancy. In some instances, however, states have included the names of individuals and organizations without finding out if they want to be listed or have experience in providing services for pregnant women. In addition, the crisis pregnancy centers and adoption agencies listed are often run by antichoice groups that provide biased counseling on abortion or other reproductive options.

WILL I HAVE TO MAKE TWO APPOINTMENTS?

In general, whether or not you will need to make two appointments depends on if you live in a state that requires a face-to-face session for the informed consent lecture or if it can be done over the phone. An increasing number of states are requiring face-to-face sessions where women must meet with a doctor in person or come to the clinic to see the lecture on videotape. However, a few do allow women to listen to a tape-recorded version of the lecture or talk with a doctor over the phone. Here's what you can expect.

Face-to-Face

If you live in a state that requires a face-to-face session or a video, you will have to make two or more appointments, depending on whether you are having a first- or second-trimester procedure. During the first appointment, pregnancy and other medical tests will be performed, and you will see the doctor or the video for the state-mandated lecture. In some states, the lecture may be given by a nurse or nurse practitioner; you will also receive the comprehensive preabortion counseling, including medical informed consent, that most clinics provide.

Note: Some clinics have been forced to raise their rates or charge an extra fee to pay doctors for the time they spend giving the state-mandated lecture. Clinics are trying to keep rate increases to a minimum; fees for the lecture range from $10 to $25.

If you are going to a clinic in another city or state, you may be able to avoid making two appointments. Some clinics have set up networks of local prochoice providers who can give you the state-mandated lecture and booklets in advance. You can also ask your own physician or another local doctor. A doctor who does not perform abortions or feels uncomfortable with the issue may make an exception for a regular patient, especially in an emergency situation. The local doctor will need to get the lecture script and booklets from the clinic and sign a special form or letter certifying that you have been given the lecture and any other required materials.

By Phone

If the lecture can be done by phone, you will hear a tape-recorded version at the time you make your appointment; or you may have to call back at another time to speak directly with a doctor. In some, but not all, cases, you will then be able to schedule an abortion for the next day. Medical tests, counseling, and the procedure will all be done at that time. Phone lectures may not be possible for all women: Face-to-face sessions, and an extra appointment, may still be required if you have a hearing disability or do not speak English (see **Waiting Periods and Other Problems,** page 27).

  While seemingly more convenient, taped lectures can cause unexpected delays. First, in states where phone lectures are allowed—Ohio, for example—women may be required to pick up the state-prepared booklets at the clinic or receive the booklets by mail at least 24 hours before an abortion. This is done so that the clinic can certify that you have had a chance to look at the booklets. You may also have to bring them with you when you go to the clinic for your appointment. If you live in another city or state, ask the clinic if you can pick up the booklets at a clinic or family planning center near you.

Some laws require longer waiting periods—2 or 3 days—when state-prepared materials are sent by mail. If you live out of state and the clinic mails the booklets to you on a Monday, you may not be able to schedule an appointment until Friday, or even the following Monday, to comply with the 24-hour requirement. In emergency situations—for instance, if delaying your appointment more than a day or two could mean a second-trimester procedure—booklets can be sent by overnight mail.

Keep in mind also that most clinics have separate tapes for first- and second-trimester abortions, and you have to hear the tape describing the procedure you are going to have. If you hear the wrong tape for any reason—for example, if you think you are in the first trimester but later find out you are in the second—the whole informed consent process will have to be repeated, and your abortion could be delayed for an additional 24 hours or longer. If you are uncertain about how long you have been pregnant, ask to hear the tapes for *both* first- and second-trimester abortions when you call to make your appointment.

WAITING PERIODS AND OTHER PROBLEMS

There is little doubt that informed consent laws have made getting an abortion more difficult and stressful for many women. Going to a clinic twice can mean extra expenses for transportation, child care, lodging, and time off work without pay, adding anywhere from $25 to $100 or more to the cost of an abortion. It may also be difficult to find a signer or translator, schedule appointments that allow you to meet your work and family obligations, or make arrangements for an overnight stay. Women under 18 may face additional restrictions and problems if they are going to a clinic in a state with a parental notification or consent law.

The following sections provide an overview of some of the practical problems informed consent laws have caused and what clinics and women are doing about them. Remember that most providers will work with you to minimize the extra time, expense, and stress these laws cause. *The earlier you call the clinic, the more time and options you will have, and the more help you are likely to get.*

Scheduling

If you live in a state where two appointments are required, you may not be able to schedule your appointments on consecutive days even if you want to. Some clinics have added extra appointment times, including evening and Saturday hours. Other are able to schedule lectures and abortions only at a few, limited times when a doctor is available. For example, even if you can go to a clinic for the state-mandated lecture on a Monday, you may not be able to make an appointment for your abortion until later in the week. In rural or small-town areas, where doctors are only at the clinic 1 or 2 days a week, delays can range from a few days to 2 weeks.

Note: If delaying your abortion even a day or two could mean you will need a second-trimester procedure, most clinics will do whatever they can to schedule your appointment as quickly as possible. Emergency waivers may be available, and state-mandated forms and booklets can be faxed or sent by overnight mail. In some instances, a doctor may be willing to give you the state-mandated lecture over the phone, even if you live in a state where face-to-face sessions are usually required.   .

Keep in mind, also, that you do *not* have to make appointments on consecutive days. For women going to a clinic in another city or state, scheduling appointments several days or even a week apart may be more convenient and less stressful. The results of any medical tests done on a first visit will remain accurate for 1 to 2 weeks, and arranging child care or time off from work may be easier, especially if you normally go shopping or run personal errands in the city or general area where the clinic is located. Combining an appointment with your weekly trip to the mall or a visit to friends could mean you won't have to come up with special, or suspicious, excuses for family, friends, or coworkers, and extra travel expenses can also be minimized (see **Chapter 6**).

Getting to the Clinic on Time

If a face-to-face session with a doctor is required, getting to the clinic on time can be vital. Many clinics do not have doctors on staff full-time, and scheduling for state-mandated lectures may be limited. If a doctor is due in surgery or has an emergency call, arriving at a clinic even a few minutes late could mean you will not be able to meet with the physician that day, and the lecture and your abortion will have to be rescheduled. To avoid unexpected delays and rescheduling, call the clinic *immediately* if you are going to be late for an appointment.

If You Have to Stay Overnight

If an overnight stay is necessary—and you can't arrange to stay with a friend—most clinics can refer you to reasonably priced, safe motels or hotels in the area. Fees vary, but you can usually get a decent room for $30 to $60 a night. You may also be able to get help from practical support networks—local prochoice groups that arrange housing, transportation, and in some cases, even child care for women who are traveling to clinics in other cities or states (see **Chapter 6**).

Travel Expenses

If you are concerned about your ability to pay for your abortion and extra travel expenses, call the clinic and ask to speak with a counselor about your financial options. You may be able to arrange a payment plan with the clinic or be eligible for a grant or an interest-free loan from an abortion assistance fund (see **Chapter 5**).

Parental Notification and Consent Laws

Most states with informed consent laws also have laws that require women under 18 to notify or get the consent of one or both parents before having an abortion, or go to court for a special hearing called a judicial bypass (see **Chapters 3 and 4**). Some, but not all, states require that your parents receive the state-mandated lecture and booklets at the same time you do. Compliance with these laws may delay your abortion by a few days, a week, or more. Your clinic will be able to tell you what you have to do to comply with the laws in your state.

Translation

In states with informed consent laws, women who have a hearing disability or who do not speak English will probably need to make two appointments: one for the state-mandated lecture—a face-to-face session is usually required even in states where phone lectures are allowed—and one for the abortion itself. A small number of clinics have staff or know translators who speak Spanish or a few Asian languages—Chinese, Vietnamese, or

Laotian, for example—but in most cases, women will need to bring in translators. Women with hearing disabilities may also be expected to bring their own signers.

WHAT THEY DON'T TELL YOU

Informed consent lectures often contain misleading information about women's ability to get welfare and child support, the risks of abortion, and when women can safely change their minds or stop a procedure. Similarly biased information on fetal development and viability may also be included in state-prepared booklets.

The following sections contain some of the facts and figures often left out of state-mandated materials. Any questions about your pregnancy and reproductive options should be answered fully and frankly by a doctor, nurse, or counselor before your procedure.

About Welfare

Under the welfare reform law signed by President Clinton in 1996, welfare benefits for single mothers and their children have been cut substantially. Individual states now determine how much you receive, how soon you have to go to work, and what other benefits you get. Specific provisions of the law that may affect women and children include a 2-year limit on benefits, a ban on benefits to legal immigrants, and a ban on additional benefits for children born while a woman is on welfare. Mandatory job training or work in low-paying jobs may also be required.

In general, whether or not a woman is eligible for welfare depends on how much she earns over an official poverty level, and the amount allowed varies from state to state. In practical terms, this means that even if you are only working part-time, you may not qualify, and even if you do, the amount of money and other benefits you receive—such as food stamps and Medicaid—could still be below official poverty levels. According to the Alan Guttmacher Institute, the average welfare payment for a single mother and child in the United States is currently about $396 per month, and in 20 states, monthly payments are under $300.

About Child Support

While federal and state efforts to track down "deadbeat dads" have attracted much media attention and political support, the reality for single mothers and their children remains pretty grim. According to figures compiled by the United States Census Bureau, only 56 percent of all single mothers receive child support, and the figure is even lower—27 percent—for single mothers who have never been married. At present, the average child support payment is $250 per month; however, only half the women receiving payments get the full amount they are due. Another 25 percent get partial payments, and 25 percent receive nothing at all.

To get child support, you may also need to establish paternity—which may mean hiring a lawyer and going to court. Getting a paternity case through court can takes weeks, or even months, and your legal fees may range from a few hundred dollars to several thousand. You can also establish paternity by contacting your local child support enforcement office and filing the necessary forms. Filing fees tend to be very low, about $25 or less, but you may still have to wait weeks or months for your case to be processed, and even then, child support payments cannot be guaranteed.

About Abortion and the Risk of Breast Cancer

Most major medical and cancer organizations have issued statements countering antichoice claims that abortion increases a woman's risk for breast cancer or that women who have abortions get a deadlier form of cancer. A recent fact sheet on abortion and breast cancer from the National Cancer Institute states:

> The available data on the relationship between induced abortions . . . and breast cancer are inconsistent and inconclusive. . . . No study [has] been found that directly links induced abortion with a deadlier form of breast cancer. In addition, the scientific rationale for an association between abortion and breast cancer is based on limited experimental data in rats, and is not consistent with human data. There is no evidence of a direct relationship between breast cancer and induced abortion.

Similar statements have been made by the National Breast Cancer Coalition, the American Cancer Society, the American College of Obstetrics and Gynecology, the American Medical Association, and the U.S. Department of Health and Human Services.

Over 30 studies have now been done on possible links between abortion and breast cancer. About half have found *no* connection, and two—including a study in Sweden that followed 49,000 women for 20 years—have concluded that abortion may actually *reduce* a woman's risk for breast cancer. Where a link between abortion and breast cancer has been found, some researchers have stated that the studies may be flawed and additional research is needed.

About Withdrawing Consent

Antichoice statements that a woman can tell a doctor to stop an abortion at any time during the procedure are inaccurate and potentially dangerous. *Once an abortion has been started, stopping the procedure can cause serious complications.* Women with retained tissue from an incomplete abortion could require additional surgery or even a hysterectomy. Other complications include abnormal bleeding, lacerations of the cervix or uterus, perforation of the uterus, or infection.

In some instances, an abortion can be stopped so long as the doctor has not begun to empty the uterus. Specifically, if you are having a second-trimester abortion, and laminaria—match-sized sticks of dried seaweed that absorb moisture and expand slowly—are being used to dilate the cervix, you may be able to change your mind after the laminaria have been inserted but before the abortion procedure itself. Depending on how long you have been pregnant and how many laminaria have been used, stopping an abortion at this point can cause an infection or a miscarriage. However, in some cases, a doctor may be able to remove the laminaria without disrupting your pregnancy or causing other complications.

No doctor or clinic will, or should, perform an abortion for a woman who has not received counseling and given her full informed consent to the procedure. At most clinics, this means that you will be asked to sign a form that says you understand the abortion procedure and its risks and are giving the doctor permission to terminate your pregnancy (see **Appendix 3**). If a woman appears upset or ambivalent about her decision or says she is being forced to have an abortion—for example, by a boyfriend who is threatening to leave her—most providers will delay the procedure and recommend additional counseling (see **Chapter 9**).

About Fetal Development and Survival

The details of fetal development are often the focus of state-prepared informed consent booklets. But just because the fetus's heartbeat or brain waves can be detected does not mean that the fetus is viable or can survive outside the womb. In fact, despite recent advances in medical technology, the point in pregnancy when a fetus is viable has *not* changed significantly in recent years. Viability varies from pregnancy to pregnancy but usually occurs at 24 to 28 weeks. Before this time, vital organs such as the lungs and kidneys are simply not developed enough. Chances of survival outside the womb at 24 weeks are only about 3 percent; survival rates at 25 to 26 weeks are 24 percent. However, intensive medical care costing thousands of dollars a day may be required, and 75 percent of the babies born at this time will have major physical or developmental disabilities.

In the United States today, approximately 99 percent of all abortions are performed in the first half of pregnancy—well before viability—and 88 percent are done in the first 12 weeks, when there is no chance whatsoever of survival outside the womb. Less than .05 percent of all abortions are performed after the 26th week. These procedures are done primarily in cases of fetal anomaly—where the fetus is so deformed, it would not survive outside the womb—or because continuing the pregnancy would endanger the woman's life or health (see **Chapter 11**).

WHAT WOMEN SAY ABOUT INFORMED CONSENT LAWS

According to providers, women's reactions to informed consent laws vary widely. While some women are angry, frustrated, or simply resigned to complying with the laws, others have found that going to a clinic for an extra appointment actually helps them feel more comfortable and confident about their abortion decision. The one thing informed consent laws haven't done is to make women change their minds or prevent them from having abortions.

The following sections contain comments and stories from providers and women who have had abortions in states with informed consent laws. Keep in mind that women's abortion experiences and reactions to informed consent laws will be different, and when you get to the clinic, you will have time to meet with a counselor privately and talk about your feelings about the laws in your state or your abortion in general.

About State-Mandated Lectures

For the most part, women do not like state-mandated lectures, and in some cases, they hardly listen to the doctor who's giving the lecture.

Melissa was in her early twenties when she had an abortion. She had to make two appointments, and take 2 days off work without pay, to terminate an unplanned pregnancy. The day she went to the clinic for her first appointment, she was more nervous about the abortion procedure itself than the videotaped lecture she had to watch.

You know, you're scared to death wondering what's going to happen to you, and you're watching this video of some guy talking to you. It's stupid. You sit there and watch the video, and I remember not paying attention to it. I don't think I even heard it.

Teresa was in college and living in a state that allowed lectures to be done by phone when she became pregnant and decided to have an abortion. She recalls that listening to the taped lecture was a minor inconvenience—much less difficult than getting to the clinic for an 8 A.M. appointment and having to explain to her parents why she and a girlfriend had to leave home for a shopping trip at 6 in the morning.

When I listened to the tape, what I heard was a really boring male doctor, totally monotone, describing the procedure and the risks. I was really surprised because I thought it was going to be totally antichoice, but it wasn't. When I got to the clinic, I had to fill out a form, and there was a space I could mark to receive the booklets, but I said, no need for that.

Tanya was married and in the second trimester of a planned pregnancy when she found out she was carrying a severely deformed fetus. She and her husband decided to have an abortion. The nearest clinic that could perform the procedure was in a state with an informed consent law, and even though they tried to get an emergency waiver, Tanya was still required to receive the state-mandated lecture and booklets. Going to the clinic for the lecture was, she recalls, "horrible."

I had to wait with other women, who were terminating healthy pregnancies, for a doctor to come in to give us the informed consent lecture, which is extremely condescending. He says things like, "You understand that the procedure you're about to get is an abortion, that you are ending your pregnancy." Then the booklet was handed out to every woman. I felt like it was being forced on me. It was really insulting because the assumption is that you're terminating a healthy pregnancy. I felt our dignity was taken away from us; we were purposely humiliated.

About Booklets

Like the lectures, state-prepared booklets on fetal development have had little impact on women's abortion decisions, and few women even ask to see them. Dale Steinberg, a provider in Pennsylvania, says that in the first 7 weeks of her state's informed consent law, her clinic performed an average of 75 abortions per week, over 500 total. During that time, only six women asked to see the state-prepared materials.

For those who do decide to look at the booklets, the pictures and descriptions of fetal development can be upsetting but rarely cause women to change their minds. An informal survey conducted by a clinic in Ohio found that 8 out of 10 women who looked at state-prepared materials said it had *no effect on their decision;* 2 out of 10 said that looking at the fetal development booklet was upsetting or made it harder for them to come to a decision, but it did *not* change their minds.

Suzy was 16 years old and 13 weeks pregnant when she had an abortion in a state with both informed consent and parental consent laws. After going to court for a judicial bypass and hearing the state-mandated lecture, she decided to look at the booklet on fetal development.

> I looked through it with the doctor in her office, and I wanted to take it with me. I was curious about it; how big this being was. At first it kind of hit me. Yeah, it looks like a baby. But then I had to weigh my choices. I knew this was a decision for me. I really couldn't raise a child.

About Going to the Clinic Twice

What women like least about informed consent laws is the 24-hour waiting period and having to go to the clinic twice. Deciding to terminate a pregnancy can be difficult, and that makes waiting periods, and the delays and other problems they cause, even more stressful and frustrating.

"Some women get really irritated," says Deni Thurman-Eyer, director of a clinic in Pennsylvania. "They understand how insulting the law is to them as responsible adult women, and they get angry. They say, 'This is the hardest thing I've ever had to deal with. I've made my decision. Why do I have to wait?'"

Thurman-Eyer and other providers note, however, that for some women, having to make an extra appointment may have unexpected benefits. Women who are scared or nervous about going to a clinic get a chance to meet clinic staff and receive extra counseling, and they often feel more relaxed and confident when they return for the procedure.

"Patients come to us, and often they don't know what to expect," says Robin Rothrock of Louisiana, one of the states with both informed consent and parental consent laws. "They're often rural women walking into an abortion clinic for the first time, and they may have misgivings, not so much about what they're doing but about how they're going to be treated.

Is it going to be 'back alley' or will they be judged? And because we work hard at providing extraordinary care, they bond with us. During the first appointment, they get all their questions answered, they get a little extra pampering, and they're pleased with the service. So when they come back for the procedure, they already know us, and they're very comfortable."

MISDIRECTED ANGER

Despite providers' best efforts, some women may still feel angry or frustrated about informed consent laws when they come to a clinic, and they may express, or act out, these negative feelings by being uncooperative or getting mad at clinic staff. While often understandable, such misdirected anger can make your appointment longer and more difficult and increase your risk of postabortion complications (see **Chapter 9**).

If you are upset or angry for any reason when you arrive at a clinic, ask to speak with a counselor. Keep in mind also that antichoice groups and legislators are the ones to blame for informed consent laws—not clinics! In fact, prochoice providers have always opposed these laws, and many doctors and clinics have worked against them by testifying, lobbying, and going to court to prevent their enactment.

INFORMED CONSENT LAWS AND WAITING PERIODS: AT A GLANCE

- Prochoice clinics have always provided **medical informed consent counseling** to ensure that women understand all their reproductive options. **Informed consent laws** are measures passed by antichoice legislators who want to make women feel scared or guilty about having abortions and make the procedure harder and more expensive to get.

- Currently in force in 11 states, informed consent laws require women to hear a state-mandated lecture 24 hours before having an abortion and be offered state-prepared materials on fetal development and medical and social services for pregnant women.

- Some informed consent laws have emergency provisions that allow the state-mandated lecture and waiting period to be waived. A waiver may be granted if you are having an abortion because of a fetal anomaly, if the pregnancy is the result of rape or incest, or if you have a violent partner or parent and coming to the clinic twice could put you at risk for physical abuse.

+ State-mandated lectures usually include information on the abortion procedure, the risks and benefits of abortion and childbirth, how long you have been pregnant, and the name of the doctor who will perform the procedure. You may also be given misleading information on the link between abortion and breast cancer, whether you will be able to get welfare and child support, and when and if you can change your mind and stop the procedure.

+ If you live in a state where a face-to-face session with a doctor is required for the state-mandated lecture, you will probably have to make two appointments. If you can listen to a tape-recorded version over the phone, only one appointment may be needed.

+ State-prepared booklets on fetal development usually contain pictures and descriptions of embryos and fetuses at 2-week intervals from 4 to 40 weeks of gestation. The booklets tend to focus on emotionally charged details of fetal growth—for example, when fingernails and toenails develop—rather than providing accurate information on fetal viability.

+ In most cases—the exception is Utah—*you do not have to read or look at state-prepared booklets if you don't want to.* Looking at the booklets may be upsetting to some women, but it does not change their minds.

+ Waiting periods can delay your abortion 1 or 2 days, a week, or longer; extra travel expenses can add anywhere from $25 to $100 or more to the cost of your abortion. Your clinic will work with you to minimize delays and other problems. *The sooner you call, the more time and options you will have.*

+ If you are under 18 and live in a state with an informed consent and a parental notification or consent law, you will have to comply with both laws before getting an abortion.

+ If you are angry or upset about informed consent laws, *don't blame the clinic!* Remember, the laws were passed by antichoice legislators. Prochoice doctors and clinics have done everything they can to oppose the laws and minimize the delays and other problems they cause.

3

PARENTAL

NOTIFICATION

AND CONSENT

LAWS

Read this chapter if you are under 18 and are going to a clinic in a state with a parental notification or consent law. To find out the law in your state, check the listings in **Appendix 1.**

Parental notification and consent laws are now in force in 31 states. The specific provisions of these laws vary widely from state to state, but in general they require minors—young women under the age of 18—to notify or get the consent of one or both parents or a legal guardian before having an abortion. If a minor cannot or does not want to involve her parents, in most cases she can go to court for a special hearing called a judicial bypass (see **Chapter 4**). At the hearing, a judge will decide if she is mature and well informed enough to make her own decision or if having an abortion is in her best interest.

Intended supposedly to "improve communication" between parents and their daughters, notification and consent laws have in fact caused much fear and confusion among young women and made it much more difficult and stressful for them to get abortions. In some states, minors whose parents are divorced or no longer live together may have to notify or get the consent of a mother or father they have not seen or talked with in years. Normally honest young women must lie or forge notes to get out of school for clinic appointments or bypass hearings. In some areas where judges deny all bypass requests or simply refuse to hear the cases, minors who cannot tell their parents are routinely advised to find a clinic out of state (see **Going out of State,** page 55).

Like informed consent laws, parental involvement laws are largely unjust and unnecessary—and create many more problems than they solve. In most states, minors already have confidential access to certain kinds of medical care—such as birth control and treatment for sexually transmitted diseases—and parental notification or consent is not needed for a young woman to give up a child for adoption. In addition, according to the Alan Guttmacher Institute, about 50 percent of all pregnant teens tell at least one parent, and others often ask for help from another responsible adult, such as an older sister, aunt, teacher, or boyfriend's parent.

If you live in a state with a parental notification or consent law, your clinic will be able to tell you what you have to do to comply with the law and help you minimize any problems or delays. Counselors can talk with you about the pros and cons of telling your parents, or another adult, and some of the things you may or may not want to say. Information and referrals are also available for teens going to court or out of state (see **Chapter 4**).

This chapter contains basic information on parental notification and consent laws, including:

- The difference between notification, consent, and mandatory counseling laws

- Why you should call a clinic as soon as you think you are pregnant—and why some teens delay making that first call

- Deciding who to talk with about your pregnancy—and what some teens say about telling their parents

- What you will need to do to comply with a notification or consent law if your parents come with you to the clinic

- What you will need to do to comply with the law if they don't come with you

THE LAWS

Some young people believe mistakenly that parental notification and consent laws make abortion illegal. *This is completely untrue!* For many young women, the parental involvement laws in force across the United States may feel like an obstacle course of different provisions and requirements, but they do *not* make abortion illegal.

What you have to do to comply with the law in your state depends on whether it requires the notification or consent of one or both parents and how loosely or strictly the clinic you go to interprets the law's provisions. For example, if your parents are coming with you to the clinic, in some cases they may have to sign a number of forms and bring several kinds of identification, including their driver's license and divorce and custody papers. At other clinics, parental ID may not even be checked. In general, here's what the laws say.

Consent Laws

If you live in a state with a parental **consent** law, one or both of your parents or a legal guardian will have to sign a form stating that you have their permission for the abortion. In most cases, clinics have interpreted consent laws to mean that one or both parents must come to the clinic with you and sign the forms there. If your parents do not come to the clinic, the form will have to be signed and notarized and given to your provider at the time of your appointment.

Note: To have a form notarized, it must be signed in the presence of a person who is certified as a notary public. You can usually find a notary at a local bank or real estate office, and some clinics now have a notary on staff. Notaries are also listed in the Yellow Pages. If you are going to a clinic in another city or state, it doesn't matter where you get the forms notarized. A small fee, a few dollars at most, may be charged for having a document notarized. In addition, notaries do not have to see the document they are notarizing, only the signature. If you are concerned about the notary or anyone else seeing a notification or consent form, you can cover the document so only the signature is visible and still get it notarized.

Notification Laws

If you live in a state with a **notification** law, your parents must be told ahead of time that you are going to have an abortion, but you will *not* need their permission. Many notification laws also include **waiting periods,** which means that even after notification occurs, you may have to wait an additional 24 to 48 hours before an abortion can be performed.

Requirements for how parents can be notified vary from state to state and clinic to clinic. Parents can sign or be mailed a notification form, or in some cases, they can be notified by phone. Again, where a signed notification form is required by state law or an individual clinic, it may have to be notarized if you are not bringing a parent with you to the clinic.

Note: While most parental notification laws state that as long as one or both parents are properly notified, minors do not need their permission for an abortion, in practice, notification often does mean consent. If your parents tell a doctor or clinic that you do not have their permission for an abortion, the clinic probably will not perform the procedure, even if you have complied with other provisions of the law. If you think your parents will not consent to your abortion or might try to stop the procedure, you may want to talk with your clinic about going to court for a judicial by-pass or finding a clinic in a state without parental involvement laws.

Mandatory Counseling Laws

A few states have passed laws that simply require minors to receive counseling on their reproductive options and have a responsible adult come with them to the clinic. Depending on the state you live in, the adult who comes with you may have to be over 21 or over 25 and can be anyone you feel comfortable with, for example, a teacher, family friend, or older sister. In most cases, the counseling you receive will be the same as the preabortion counseling provided by most clinics. You will be given information on all your reproductive options, including carrying the pregnancy to term and adoption, and a description of the abortion procedure and its risks (see **Chapter 9**).

Note: Mandatory counseling laws are different from so-called informed consent laws, which require women to receive state-mandated lectures and printed materials before having an abortion. If you live in a state with an informed consent law and a parental involvement law, you will have to comply with both laws. This means you will have to receive the state-mandated lecture for the informed consent law, plus any preabortion counseling required for the parental involvement law. Medical informed consent counseling at the clinic may also be required (see **Chapter 2**).

Clinic Requirements

Even if a state has no parental involvement law, some providers may require minors to have a parent or other adult come with them to the clinic or sign a consent form. In general, a provider is more likely to require parental or adult involvement if you are under 16 or driving long distances to a clinic in another city or state. In such instances, adult involvement is often requested to ensure that you are not alone after the procedure and and that you call the clinic immediately if any complications develop. You will also not be allowed to leave the clinic alone or drive yourself home if your abortion is done with extra pain medication or a sedative or if you are having laminaria inserted (see **Chapter 9**).

EXCEPTIONS TO THE LAWS

Most parental notification and consent laws contain special provisions that allow some minors to have abortions without telling a parent. Exceptions to the laws vary from state to state, and individual doctors and clinics may interpret these provisions differently. Your provider will be able to tell you if you are eligible to waive the parental notification and consent requirement in your state and how to do it.

Judicial Bypass

Most parental notification and consent laws have a judicial bypass provision for women under 18 who feel they cannot or do not want to tell their parents. The only states with parental involvement laws that do not have judicial or other bypass provisions are Idaho and Utah.

Keep in mind that a bypass hearing is *not* a trial, and most laws state that if a young woman is mature and well informed enough, a bypass *must* be granted. If a minor is not mature or well informed, a bypass may still be granted if the judge rules that having an abortion without telling her parents is in her best interest, for example, if the pregnancy is the result of rape or incest or if her parents are violent and could beat or abuse her. The laws also require that bypass hearings be quick, confidential, and free (see **Chapter 4**).

Emancipated Minors

Many parental involvement laws also state that a woman under 18 does not have to tell her parents or go to court for a judicial bypass if she is an emancipated minor. In general, you could be considered an emancipated minor if you are married, already have a child, or are financially independent of and living apart from your parents. The definition of emancipation varies from state to state, and some laws require all unmarried teens under 18 to comply with parental notification and consent laws, whether or not they have children or live apart from their parents.

Notification of Other Family Members

Several states have laws that allow minors to notify or get the consent of an adult family member other than their parents—for example, a grandparent, aunt or uncle, or older sister or brother. The specific provisions of these laws vary widely from state to state. In some cases, the circumstances in which another family member may be notified are extremely limited: for example, in North Carolina a minor's grandmother may be notified, but only if the teen has been living with her for 6 months. In other cases, the family member may have to go to the clinic with the young woman, sign a notification or consent form, or file a special affidavit at court.

Physician Bypass

A few states allow doctors to waive parental involvement requirements if they believe a young woman is mature and informed enough to make her own decisions. A physician bypass may also be available where a pregnancy is the result of rape or incest or if the doctor believes that telling your parents could put you at risk for physical or emotional abuse. In most cases, a special letter or form is required, and the doctor who signs it must be affiliated with the clinic. Other doctors, such as a regular gynecologist or family doctor, cannot grant a physician bypass, even if they might be willing to.

IF YOUR PARENTS ARE DIVORCED OR SEPARATED

Parental involvement laws usually require the notification or consent of one or both of a minor's *biological* parents. If your parents are divorced or separated, or you are not living with your biological parents or a legal guardian, you may still have to notify them or get their consent for the abortion—even if you have not seen or talked with them for several years.

In some states where the notification or consent of both parents is required, the laws contain special provisions for minors whose parents are divorced or no longer living together. Specifically, if your parents are separated or divorced and your mother or father has full custody, you may only need to notify or get the consent of your custodial parent. If your parents have joint custody, it is likely that both will have to sign notification or consent forms. A stepparent is usually not allowed to sign unless she or he is also your legal guardian.

If you are adopted, your adoptive parents are your legal guardians and can sign any notification or consent form for you. If you are in foster care or are a ward of the state, your foster parents or state-appointed guardian may not be able to sign the forms—state laws do not allow them to—and a judicial bypass hearing may be necessary.

CALL THE CLINIC *NOW!*

✔ While an unplanned pregnancy is a crisis for any woman, for teenagers the experience can be especially stressful and frightening, whether or not they live in a state with a parental involvement law. Providers note that teenagers are more likely to delay calling a clinic and to be near or in the second trimester when they do.

Why do so many young women delay? Fear and lack of information are the primary reasons. Young women are often unfamiliar with their bodies and menstrual cycles and may be unsure if they are pregnant—or simply afraid of finding out that they are. Teenagers are also less likely to have been to a clinic before, and many have not had a pelvic exam. They may be worried about how they are going to pay for the abortion or scared about the pain of the procedure itself. Fear of parents' disappointment and anger is another reason for delay, especially if your parents are strongly opposed to abortion or have beaten or physically or emotionally abused you in the past.

While fear and denial are common and understandable reactions to an unplanned pregnancy, *the sooner you call a clinic for a pregnancy test and counseling, the more time and options you will have.* Keep in mind that even if your parents support your decision to have an abortion, scheduling an appointment may take several days, a week, or longer. If you are in the second trimester, it may be harder to find a clinic, and the procedure will cost more.

For many young woman, calling a clinic turns out to be easier and more reassuring than they expected. Many clinics have free 800 numbers, so long-distance charges won't show up on your parents' phone bill. All calls are strictly confidential, which means the clinic will not tell anyone that you have called or made an appointment unless you say it's okay.

Note: Providers know that any surgery can be scary for young women, and many take extra steps to minimize the pain and stress of the abortion procedure for teenagers. At some clinics, abortions for women under 18 are performed with additional medication—either IV sedation or a general anesthetic—or with laminaria, a method for dilating the cervix that can reduce pain and discomfort (see **Chapter 9**). A counselor will be with you during the abortion to hold your hand or talk with you, and some clinics will even allow you to have a parent, boyfriend, or other support person with you during the procedure.

Teenagers often ask a friend, family member, or other support person to call the clinic for them, either because they are frightened or do not feel safe or comfortable making the call from home. However hard it may be to find the time and privacy you need, if at all possible, *call the clinic yourself.* Having someone else call for you can result in confusion and misinformation—for example, if a friend writes down the wrong time or address—and clinic staff will often need to speak with you directly before you can make an appointment.

Depending on the clinic, scheduling an appointment by phone can take as little as 10 to 15 minutes or over half an hour. Keep in mind that clinic lines are often busy, and it may take you several calls to schedule your appointment; or you may have to leave a name and number and have a counselor call you back. In such instances, you can often tell a provider to leave a confidential or "coded" message—just a name and phone number with no other identifying information, such as the clinic's name or why you called.

If you are concerned about making calls or getting messages at home, see if you can call from a friend's house or use her or his phone as a contact number for the clinic. In addition, some teens now have personal pagers. If you have a part-time job, you may be able to make or get calls at work.

WHO TO TELL

About 50 percent of all pregnant teens talk with their parents about their abortion decisions—whether or not they live in a state with a parental involvement law—and many others tell an adult friend or family member, such as a neighbor, teacher, or older sister or brother. Telling a parent, if at all possible, makes complying with notification and consent laws easier and less stressful. In addition, some young women, especially those 15 and under, often find they need an adult to help them with the practical details of arranging an abortion, including taking time off from school, driving to and from the clinic, and paying for the procedure.

Getting emotional support during an unplanned pregnancy, and sharing your feelings with someone, is important for all women. In general, the people you talk with should respect your confidentiality and be supportive and nonjudgmental. They should not blame you or try to make you feel bad about being pregnant or having an abortion. Instead, they should focus on your wants and needs and making sure you receive the best care possible—whatever you decide (see **Chapter 8**).

In the end, who you tell about your pregnancy and what or how much you tell them are extremely personal decisions. When choosing someone to confide in, think about what you need right now and *trust your own instincts.* Most clinics will encourage you to talk with at least one parent or supportive adult, but you are the best judge of what is and isn't possible and who you can and can't tell.

"My Folks Will Kill Me"—and Then What?

For some young women, just the thought of telling a parent about an unplanned pregnancy may be more frightening and stressful than actually doing it. Providers note that many teenagers say, "Oh, my folks will kill me," when what they really mean is that they are afraid a parent will be angry or disappointed when she or he finds out they are pregnant.

Yes, telling parents or a guardian about an unplanned pregnancy is intimidating, and there's a good chance yours may be angry or disappointed when you first tell them. After the initial upset, however, you may find that your parents support your decision to have an abortion and that their main concern is your health and well-being and making sure you go to a clinic where you get good care.

If you are uncertain about whether you want to talk with your parents about your pregnancy, make a list of pros and cons, and again, *trust your instincts.* Think about whether you have ever talked with them about sensitive or difficult subjects, like birth control, drugs and alcohol, or sexually transmitted diseases. How did they react? How do they respond when they think you are wrong or careless? Is it okay for you to disagree with them? How does a crisis or bad news affect them? What did they do when your older sister or a neighbor's teenage daughter got pregnant?

Your clinic can help you evaluate how your parents may react. Counselors will often role-play or rehearse different approaches with you and suggest specific things you may or may not want to say. Some clinics also offer free or low-cost family counseling sessions where a counselor meets with you and your parents to discuss your pregnancy and reproductive options.

What Teens Say about Telling Their Parents

Telling parents or other friends or family about an unplanned pregnancy can be difficult regardless of your age, and people's reactions may often disappoint or surprise you. In some cases, a pregnant teenager may find a parent's negative response especially depressing and frustrating (see **If You Decide Not to Tell,** page 48). In others, going through an unplanned pregnancy and abortion together may strengthen the bonds between parents and their daughters.

Tina was 17 years old and living in a state with a parental consent law when she got pregnant and told her mother she wanted to have an abortion.

> I told my mom right away. That was probably the hardest thing I had to do, telling her about it. When I first told her, she cried; she was really upset. But the next day, she came up to me and said, "I'll be there for you, and I'll do anything you need; I'll take you wherever you want to go. Whatever you want to do, I'm behind you." So it was a little hard at first, but it brought us a lot closer together. We went through the whole thing together.

Even when parents are not supportive, teenagers often find a relative or other concerned adult who they feel they can confide in or ask for help. Judy was 16 and had just broken up with an abusive boyfriend when she found out she was pregnant. When he threatened to "get her" if she had an abortion, she tried talking with her mother.

> I wasn't living with my mother at the time, and when I told her I was pregnant, she quit her job, she was so upset about me being pregnant. She wouldn't talk to me afterwards. Whenever I tried to talk with her, she was very, very cold. She would say she couldn't believe I'd gone and gotten pregnant.

While Judy eventually became reconciled with her mother, at the time she turned to a family friend who provided emotional support and drove her to the clinic.

> She and my mom were best friends, and I've always been close to her. She was supposed to be out of town the day of the abortion, but she came back the night before and surprised me. That meant a lot. She

took me to the clinic the next day, and she and her boyfriend were there for me.

Getting support from an adult—in this case her mother—was also essential for Nina, who was only 14 and living in a state with a parental notification law when she got pregnant. Telling her mother, she recalls, was "really scary and really hard."

It's difficult to tell your parents, "I messed up" or "I'm having sex," or "I'm being irresponsible," but I always had an open relationship with my mom and she knew I was sexually active at the time. She was pretty straightforward about it. I had only taken a home pregnancy test, so she said, "First we'll make sure you're really pregnant, and if you are, then we'll get it taken care of." It was really early on, like the first three weeks, and my mom set up everything for me and signed all the forms. It wasn't even considered that anything else would be an option. It felt good.

If You Decide Not to Tell

In an ideal world, all pregnant teenagers would be able to turn to their parents for help and support, but for some, this is simply not possible. Communication between parents and a teenage daughter may be so poor that any discussion of sex, let alone pregnancy and abortion, is virtually taboo. In the case of a family crisis—for example, if a parent has recently lost a job or is going through a divorce—you may decide not to tell your parents to spare them additional stress. If your parents oppose abortion, you may be afraid they will throw you out of the house or pressure you to continue the pregnancy against your will. If they are violent or abuse drugs or alcohol, you could be at increased risk for physical or emotional abuse.

If you decide not to tell your parents—whatever your reasons—most clinics will respect your decision and help you to get a judicial bypass or find a provider in a nearby state that does not have a parental involvement law. Counselors will also encourage you to get help and emotional support from other people and talk with you about how to keep your pregnancy and abortion a secret (see **Chapter 4**).

While deciding not to tell a parent may be the smartest, and safest, thing for some young women, it can also be extremely painful. Realizing that your parents may not be supportive at a time when you really need them can be upsetting, frustrating, or very depressing. You may also feel that not telling them means something is wrong with you.

However sad or angry you feel right now, keep in mind that not involv-
ing a parent is often a sign of maturity—that you are able to make and
take responsibility for your own decisions. Keeping the pregnancy and
abortion a secret may even turn out to be a positive experience. For many
young women, it may be one of the first times they make an important or
life-changing decision on their own, and they may feel more confident
and better about themselves as a result.

Support and Confidentiality—Think before You Tell

The need for support during an unplanned pregnancy must often be balanced by the need for confidentiality. Simply put, not all people will keep
your secret, even if they say they will, and you should think carefully before you tell.

For example, confiding in a teacher or school counselor can be especially risky. State laws on the reporting responsibilities of school staff are
often vague and confusing. If you tell a teacher or school counselor you
are pregnant, she or he may think telling the principal or your parents is
required by law—even though it is a clear violation of your confidentiality.

Note: In most cases, it is, in fact, *illegal* for a teacher, school counselor, or
principal to tell your parents you are pregnant or having an abortion. If
you tell any school employee you are pregnant and she or he threatens to
tell your parents, call a clinic or local chapter of the American Civil Liberties Union (ACLU) immediately (see **Appendix 2**). In some cases, you may
be able to stop the school from contacting your parents.

You may also want to think carefully before talking about your pregnancy
with schoolmates or other friends, even if they "swear" not to tell anyone.
Teen friendships, however intense, are sometimes short-lived, and the
person who has been your "best friend" for only a few weeks or months
may not be as trustworthy as you think.

Besides telling her mother she was pregnant, Nina also told two of her
friends at school. After taking a day off for the abortion, she says, she
found out they had not kept her secret.

They told everyone at school. It was really hard on me. People would
say things about me behind my back, or someone would come up to
me and say "I heard you were out of school because you got pregnant

and had an abortion." That happened about three times, and it was always a boy. It was tough because I don't think anyone knew what I had to do and what I had to go through. I was embarrassed because they had found out, and I was mad because my friends told on me.

SO YOUR PARENTS KNOW

✓ While telling your parents you are pregnant can make complying with parental notification and consent laws easier, it doesn't guarantee you won't run into some problems and delays. Again, many notification laws have 24- or 48-hour waiting periods, and if you live in a state with a

---

CONFIDENTIALITY AND ABUSE: WHEN REPORTING IS NECESSARY

While most doctors, nurses, teachers, and counselors should keep anything you tell them confidential, in some instances, they may not be able to. School administrators, medical personnel, and clinic staff are required by law to report suspected cases of child abuse or child endangerment to the proper authorities. If you tell a doctor, nurse, teacher, or counselor that you are being physically, sexually, or emotionally abused by a parent, family member, or other adult (such as a coach or employer), the person you tell will have to report it to the child protection agency in your area. Reporting may also be required in cases of alcohol or drug abuse, or any other behavior by a parent that puts you at risk for emotional or physical abuse.

While reporting abuse to a counselor or other adult can and should stop it—at least temporarily—in many cases, it may not. Reporting could mean you or the abusing parent will be taken out of the home. You could also be put in foster care or made a ward of the state, in which case you might have to go to court for a judicial bypass hearing and your abortion could be delayed by several days or weeks. For teenagers who remain at home, the abuse may continue or become worse. They may be blamed or punished for telling someone about it—or for getting pregnant or going to a clinic.

If you are being abused by a parent or other adult, call a clinic, family planning center, or rape crisis center in your area (see **Appendix 2**). Any of these agencies will be able to give you information on the reporting requirements in your state and what may or may not happen if you tell someone at a clinic or school that you are being abused.

two-parent notification or consent law, you may have to get both parents to sign all the required forms even if they are divorced or no longer living together. Clinics within the same state may also vary in how strictly or loosely they interpret a law's requirements; your provider will tell you exactly what you and your parents will and won't have to do.

Keep in mind also that even if your parents sign the forms and go with you to the clinic, having an abortion must be *your* decision. No abortion will be performed if you tell a counselor you are being forced or pressured to terminate your pregnancy or if you appear extremely upset or ambivalent about your decision. Any teenager who says she does not want to have an abortion will be offered additional counseling and referrals for prenatal care.

When Your Parents Are at the Clinic

Having a parent come with you to the clinic is probably the easiest way to comply with a notification or consent law. Required forms can be signed at the clinic, and delays and other problems kept to a minimum. In states with two-parent notification or consent laws, both parents must sign all required forms. This means that if only one parent comes with you to the clinic, you will need to bring signed forms for the other parent.

Consent and notification forms are usually short, simple documents that state either that your parents give their consent for your abortion or that they have been notified or are aware that you intend to terminate your pregnancy. Your parents may also have to sign a form stating that they are, in fact, your parents, or in the case of a guardian, that she or he is legally responsible for you (see **Appendix 3**). In states that have notification laws with waiting periods, providers may be able to mail or fax forms to you ahead of time. You and your parents can then either bring them with you to the clinic and sign them there or have them signed and notarized before your appointment.

Identification   Providers usually require teenagers and their parents or guardians to bring some form of identification with them to the clinic. In most cases, minors will need to have a birth certificate or photo ID, such as a driver's license, passport, or valid state ID. If you don't have a copy of your birth certificate or any other identification, many clinics will tell you to bring a recent school yearbook with your name and picture in it.

Parents will also need to bring a photo ID as well as other legal documents that prove they are, in fact, your parents, especially if you and your father or mother have different last names. Single or remarried parents may have to bring divorce and custody papers, and legal guardians will need to have papers that show proof of guardianship.

In cases where legal proof of custody is not available, parents or guardians may need to bring other documents that prove they are legally responsible for you, such as an insurance form that shows you are covered by their plan. If you live in a state with a two-parent notification or consent law and one of your biological parents is dead, you may also need to bring a copy of the deceased parent's death certificate.

At present, clinics vary widely in how strictly they enforce ID requirements for parents. In some cases, the parent or other adult coming with you to the clinic will only be asked to sign a form stating that she or he is your parent. No ID or other documentation will be required unless it is clearly obvious that the adult is not your parent.

Counseling   Parental involvement laws and clinic policy also vary widely on whether or not parents can or are required to participate in preabortion counseling sessions. In some cases, your parents will have to receive preabortion counseling or state-mandated informed consent materials with you (see **Chapter 2**). In others, some kind of counseling for parents—either with you or alone—may be available, but not mandatory, and you will be in control of what happens during the appointment. For example, your parents may not be allowed in the room during your counseling session unless you say it's okay. Separate counseling sessions for parents and teenagers can also be arranged in different parts of the building, and at some clinics, separate counseling may not be offered without your permission.

In general, counseling sessions for parents are similar to the preabortion counseling you receive. Your parents or guardian will be given information on the abortion procedure and its risks, and a counselor will talk with them about any questions or concerns they may have. Separate counseling sessions will also be confidential. No information from your current or previous counseling sessions will be discussed with your parents.

Even if your parents are required to receive preabortion counseling with you, you will still meet with a counselor privately, and that session will also be confidential. Complete confidentiality will not be possible, however, if you tell your counselor, or any clinic staff, that you are being pressured to have an abortion or that you are still unsure about your decision. In such cases, if your parents are with you at the clinic, they will be asked to join the counseling session, and your counselor will help you tell them that you do not want to have an abortion at this time.

Note: Most clinics are also sensitive to any signs of an inappropriate relationship between a teenager and her parents; for example, a mother or father who insists on being with their daughter at all times during an appointment or who does not let her speak for herself during a counseling session. In such instances, counselors will make sure they talk with the young woman in private to find out if she is currently at risk for physical or emotional abuse or is being pressured to have an abortion if she doesn't want to.

When Your Parents Aren't at the Clinic

If your parents do not come with you to the clinic, what you will need to do to comply with the parental involvement law in your state will depend on whether the law requires consent or notification. If you live in a state with a consent law, your provider will give you the consent forms your parents need to sign—forms can usually be picked up at the clinic or mailed to you—and you will have to bring the signed forms with you when you go to the clinic for your appointment. In general, the forms will have to be notarized, or the clinic may require that you bring copies of your parent's identification, such as a driver's license or divorce and custody papers.

Notification laws, on the other hand, usually provide several options for compliance when a minor's parents are not coming with her to the clinic. Again, you can bring signed, notarized forms with you at the time of your appointment, or your provider may be able to notify your parents by phone or mail. If notification is done by phone, a doctor or counselor at the clinic will call your parents and tell them you are going to have an abortion. If notification is done by mail, the clinic sends a letter, often by registered or certified mail. This means that the provider will receive notification from the post office that your parents received the letter, but a signed notification form will not be required when you come to the clinic for your appointment.

Keep in mind that notification by phone or mail—while sometimes less complicated and stressful—can cause additional delays in scheduling an abortion, especially if the law in your state includes a 24- or 48-hour waiting period. For example, your appointment could have to be rescheduled—in some cases more than once—if notification is done by phone and your parents are not available when the clinic calls. When notification is done by mail, clinics may add a day or two to the waiting period to make sure your parents have received the letter. For instance, if the clinic mails a notification letter on a Monday, you might not be able to schedule an appointment until Thursday or Friday, even if the law in your state only requires a 24-hour waiting period.

If Your Parents Are Divorced or Separated

Parental involvement laws that require the notification or consent of both parents may contain special provisions for minors whose parents are divorced or separated. If one of your parents has full custody, notification or consent forms may only have to be signed by the custodial parent. Similarly, if you live in a state with a two-parent notification law and are no longer in touch with an absent or noncustodial parent, the clinic may only need to mail a letter to the parent's last known address.

Unfortunately, some laws still require the notification or consent of both parents, whether or not they are divorced or still living together, and in cases where a teenager can or only wants to get one parent to sign forms, a judicial bypass hearing may be necessary. For instance, if a young woman's parents are divorced and her father opposes abortion, she and her mother may decide they do not want to ask him to sign a notification or consent form. In such cases—and especially if going to a clinic in another state is not an option—a judicial bypass hearing would be required, and the teen's mother may have to go to court with her.

Mandatory Counseling and Other Alternatives to Parental Involvement

If you live in a state with a mandatory counseling law, a form stating that you have received the preabortion counseling required by the law will have to be signed by a family member or other responsible adult who is, depending on the state, over 21 or over 25. In some cases, the counselor you go to for the session will have to be someone who is not employed by the clinic—such as a teacher, family planning counselor, minister, or rabbi—and the adult who comes with you and signs the form will have to be present during the counseling session.

If the counseling must be provided by someone not affiliated with the clinic, you will be given information on the professionals in your community you can speak with—such as nurses, teachers, and clergy—and referrals to specific individuals may also be available. In emergencies—for example, if you are near the second trimester and can't arrange a counseling session or find an adult to come with you the day of the appointment—a clinic may be able to arrange a counseling session for you, and a staff member will sign the required forms. In most instances, the counseling you receive will be similar to the preabortion counseling provided to all women at prochoice clinics.

If you live in a state where the notification or consent of another family member is allowed, the person you tell—grandparent, aunt, or brother—will probably have to sign a form similar to the notification or consent forms a parent signs. In addition, the forms may have to be notarized, or appropriate identification provided, depending on whether the family member signing for you does or does not come to the clinic.

GOING OUT OF STATE

For many young women who cannot tell their parents, going out of state may be easier than going to court for a judicial bypass hearing, even if the nearest clinic is several hours away. In Massachusetts, which has had a two-parent consent law since 1981, it is estimated that one-third of all teenagers seeking abortions go out of state—about 1,200 per year. Similarly, in some parts of Louisiana, requests for judicial bypass are routinely turned down, and teenagers who cannot tell their parents are referred to providers in Texas or Arkansas.

If you decide to go out of state, your clinic will refer you to providers in the nearest state or states that have no parental involvement laws, and in some cases, you may be able to call an out-of-state provider and make an appointment before you leave the clinic. Your counselor may also talk with you about the practical details of going out of state, such as finding someone to drive you to the clinic, getting out of school, and what you will need to tell parents and friends to protect your confidentiality (see **Chapter 6**).

As more and more states pass parental involvement laws, many teens—especially those in the South and Midwest—are finding that the states nearest them also have some kind of notification or consent law in force. Getting an abortion in another state may still be easier, for example, if you live in a state with a two-parent consent law and a neighboring state only requires the notification of one parent.

PARENTAL NOTIFICATION AND CONSENT LAWS: AT A GLANCE

• Now in force in 31 states, parental notification and consent laws require women under the age of 18 to notify one or both parents or get their consent before having an abortion. If you don't want to tell your parents, you can get a waiver or bypass by going to court for a special hearing.

• *Don't delay in calling a clinic!* The sooner you get a pregnancy test and counseling, the more time and options you will have.

• If you live in a state with a parental **consent** law, one or both of your parents will have to sign a form that says you have their permission to get an abortion. If your parents do not come with you to the clinic and sign the form there, you may have to have the form notarized.

• If you live in a state with a parental **notification** law, one or both of your parents will have to be told 24 to 48 hours ahead of time that you are having an abortion. Your parents may have to sign a form at the clinic; in some states, notification can occur by phone or mail.

• If you live in a state with a **mandatory counseling** law, you will have to receive special counseling on your reproductive options, and a family member or adult over 21 or over 25 will have to sign a form stating you have received the counseling.

• You may not have to tell your parents if you are an emancipated minor or live in a state that allows other family members—such as a grandparent, aunt, or older brother or sister—to sign notification or consent forms for you. Some states also allow doctors to sign a special bypass form stating you are mature and informed enough to make your own decision.

• For some teenagers, going out of state may be easier than telling their parents or going to court for a judicial bypass hearing. If this is the case, your clinic will refer you to a provider in a nearby state that does not have a parental involvement law.

• You are the best judge of whether or not to tell your parents, or anybody else, about your pregnancy and abortion. *Trust your instincts!*

• Getting support during an unplanned pregnancy is important, but think carefully about who you tell and ask for help. If you tell school or clinic staff that you are being sexually, physically, or emotionally abused, they *must* report it to a child protection agency.

• Find out exactly what you have to do to comply with the parental notification or consent law in your state. Ask your provider what forms you or your parents have to sign, whether they have to be notarized, and what forms of identification you need to bring with you to the clinic.

♦ Even if your parents sign all the forms and come with you to the clinic, having an abortion must be *your* decision. If you tell a counselor that you do not want to have an abortion, the procedure will be postponed and you and your parents will be offered additional counseling.

4

WHEN YOU CAN'T TELL YOUR PARENTS: THE JUDICIAL BYPASS

Read this chapter if you live in a state with a parental notification or consent law and have decided you want to go to court for a judicial bypass hearing or are just thinking about it. To find out the law in your state, check the listings in **Appendix 1.**

Of the 31 states with parental notification or consent laws currently in force, 26 allow **judicial bypass hearings** for minors—women under 18—who cannot or do not want to tell their parents they are pregnant. The hearing is *not* a trial, and going to court does *not* mean you are asking the judge for permission to have an abortion. Rather, most laws state that a bypass must be granted if a minor is mature and well informed enough to make her own decision or if having an abortion is in her best interest—for example, if the pregnancy is caused by rape or incest or her parents have physically abused her.

In addition, judicial bypass hearings must be *quick, free, and confidential.* Hearings usually last about 10 to 30 minutes, and in most cases, a court-appointed lawyer, also free, will be with you. The only other people allowed in the room will be the judge, a court clerk or court reporter, and, in some cases, a court-appointed psychologist or social worker. After the hearing, all records of the case will be sealed—no one will be allowed to see them—and in some states, records are destroyed after a period of several years.

However easy and unintimidating the laws make it seem, for many teenagers going to court can feel frightening, overwhelming, or just impossible. Scheduling a hearing can delay an abortion by several days or weeks, and in some states, antichoice judges turn down all bypass requests or simply refuse to hear the cases.

Fortunately, in many states today, clinics and prochoice lawyers are working together to make sure that any young woman who decides to go to court will get the information and support she needs. When you call a clinic, you will receive instructions on how to arrange a hearing, referrals to prochoice lawyers or the court officials you will need to speak with, and counseling on what to wear and how to act in court. Clinic staff and lawyers may also help you fill out forms, make phone calls, and give you advice on how to answer any questions you may be asked during the hearing.

This chapter contains basic information on how to arrange and prepare for a judicial bypass hearing. The material covered includes:

♦ How, and how long it takes, to schedule a hearing

♦ Whether you will have to receive special counseling or talk with a court-appointed psychologist or social worker before the hearing

♦ What to wear and how to act in court

♦ The questions you may be asked at the hearing, and what to do if a judge says anything that makes you angry or upset

♦ What happens if the judge says no

HOW TO ARRANGE A HEARING

For many teens who decide to go to court, the first step is calling a clinic. Judicial bypass provisions vary from state to state and county to county, and your clinic will be able to tell you exactly what you have to do to arrange a hearing in your area. In some cases, you may be referred directly to a prochoice attorney who will help you schedule a hearing; in others, scheduling is done through the clinic or directly at the courthouse.

Note: A few providers—such as private doctors with small practices—refuse to see minors who have decided to go to court. If you are unable to find a clinic that can give you information on judicial bypass procedures in your area, call the National Abortion Federation referral line at 800-772-9100 or the Planned Parenthood referral line at 800-230-7526.

Arranging a hearing can take several days, a week, or longer, so the sooner you call a clinic, the more time and options you will have.

Getting a Lawyer

Most parental involvement laws state that any minor going to court for a bypass hearing is entitled to a free, court-appointed lawyer. If you need an attorney, in most cases you will be referred to one either by your clinic or a court official, and *you will not have to pay any lawyer's fees.* Attorneys on clinic and court referral lists are usually prochoice lawyers who are familiar with judicial bypass procedures—and the different judges—in their areas and will be able to minimize any delays and other problems going to court may cause.

Bypass procedures—and whether or not you will need a lawyer for your hearing—vary widely from state to state and court to court. In most states, having a lawyer is necessary; in a few, hearings are very informal— you will talk with the judge for a few minutes—and an attorney is not required. Similarly, in some cases, you will meet with your attorney before the hearing, and she or he will give you detailed information about what will be happening in court and the kinds of questions you may be asked; in others, the only time you will see your lawyer will be at the hearing itself.

Filing a Petition

To arrange a judicial bypass hearing, you have to file (submit) a petition with the court. In most cases, the bypass petition is a short legal form that states you are under 18, pregnant, and want to have an abortion without telling your parents (see **Appendix 3**). A counselor or lawyer may help you fill out the form or file it for you; or you may have to go to the courthouse and file the petition with the clerk of the court—the court official who will schedule the hearing and tell you, or your lawyer or counselor, where and when it will be.

Filing a petition is free—you will *not* have to pay any court costs—and any forms you file for the hearing will be strictly confidential. In some cases, your name, address, and any other identifying information will not appear on the petition or any other court documents related to your case; the petition will be filed in the name of Jane Doe or simply left blank. In other instances, personal information will be required when you fill out the petition or other forms, but these documents will be sealed after the hearing.

Parental notification and consent laws also specify where petitions must be filed—which court or county—and your clinic or lawyer will give you instructions or help you to make sure you file the forms in the right place. In general, petitions are filed and bypass hearings held either in district, juvenile, or family law courts—called probate or chancery courts in some states—in the county where you live or where the clinic is located.

Since many laws state that individual counties can set their own bypass procedures, where you file can make a difference, and your clinic or lawyer will usually have you file the petition in the county where you are least likely to encounter any problems or delays. If you have a choice—and especially if you live in a small town or rural area or are concerned about running into someone you know at court—it is probably better to have the hearing in the county where the clinic is located. Judges and courts in these areas usually have more experience with judicial bypass procedures and are more likely to conduct hearings quickly and fairly, even in cases where a judge is personally opposed to abortion or feels uncomfortable with the issue.

Judges and court personnel in small towns and rural areas—where few clinics are located—do hearings less frequently and may be less evenhanded in their treatment of these cases and pregnant teens. In rural districts some judges simply deny all bypass requests or refuse to hear the cases. Minors calling courts to arrange a hearing may also be given false or misleading information; for example, you might be told you will have to hire an attorney or pay your own court and legal fees.

Note: The U.S. Supreme Court has ruled that all parental notification and consent laws must contain a bypass provision of some sort. This means that *going to court is your right.* If you call a court and are told you cannot have a hearing, *don't give up!* Call your clinic and ask for help and further instructions. Legal advice and referrals to prochoice lawyers may also be available from a local office of the American Civil Liberties Union (see **Appendix 2**). In addition, if your request for a bypass is denied, you can refile or appeal.

If going to court in the county where you live or where the clinic is located is not possible, other options may still be available. In some states, hearings can be held in any county that is next to the one where the young woman is living or where the clinic is located; others allow hearings in any county where the teenager "is found," which basically means any county in the state.

Even if you live in a state where the law says hearings can only be held in the county where you live, you may still be able to move the hearing to another county by filing a petition called a change of venue. Your clinic or lawyer will be able to tell you if a change of venue is possible and help you file the appropriate papers. A request for a change of venue may take a day or two to process, but in emergency situations, it can be done in under 24 hours.

How Long It Takes

In general, once a petition is filed, a hearing must be held within a specific period of time. Depending on where you live, this may be anywhere from 24 hours to 5 days. Again, how the laws are interpreted varies widely from state to state and court to court, and delays can occur. In some cases, a hearing can be scheduled for the same day a petition is filed; in others, you will have to wait several days or even a week.

Delays are especially likely if you live in a state where the time between filing a petition and scheduling a hearing is measured in business or working days, rather than calendar days, which means weekends and holidays are not included. For example, if you live in a state where a hearing must be scheduled within 5 working days, you could file a petition on a Tuesday and the hearing would not have to be scheduled until the following Tuesday—5 days plus the weekend.

Going to court also means you may have to take time off from school. Although some clinics routinely arrange hearings and abortions for the same day, in other cases, this may not be possible. While some laws state that hearings should be scheduled so students do not have to miss classes, most courts are only open during school hours, Monday through Friday, 9 A.M. to 4 or 4:30 P.M. Meetings with counselors and lawyers may also have to be scheduled for the day of the hearing, and you may need to take an afternoon or a whole day off just to go to court.

Once you get to court, hearings may also be delayed simply because a judge is not available. Bypass hearings are often squeezed in during breaks in a judge's regular schedule—such as a trial recess or lunch hour—and teens and their lawyers may have to wait anywhere from 30 minutes to 2 hours or longer. In emergency situations—for example, if going to court and the clinic on different days could mean your parents will find out—delays can be minimized. You may be able to arrange a hearing for first thing in the morning and go directly from court to the clinic for your abortion.

Precourt Counseling and Interviews

In some states, minors are required to receive additional counseling on their reproductive options or have an interview with a court-appointed psychologist or social worker before their hearing. If this is the case, your clinic or attorney will tell you how to arrange these sessions and what will happen when you meet with the counselor, psychologist, or social worker.

In general, counseling on reproductive options will be similar to the preabortion counseling most clinics provide for all women. A counselor will make sure you understand all your reproductive options, including carrying the pregnancy to term and adoption, and will give you information on the abortion procedure and its risks (see **Chapter 9**). In some cases, you will be able to receive the counseling at the clinic where you are going to have your abortion. In other cases, you may have to go to a family planning center or to another group or individual who is not associated with the clinic.

Note: The judge at your hearing may ask detailed questions about your pregnancy and the abortion procedure, so you should be sure you understand all the information you are given during any precourt counseling sessions. Remember that counselors or other clinic staff will answer any questions you may have, and a sonogram or pelvic exam may be performed before you go to court so you will know exactly how long you have been pregnant. If you are given any written materials at the clinic, reviewing them the night before the hearing may also help you feel better prepared for any questions the judge may ask.

Interviews with court-appointed psychologists or social workers are usually intended to provide the judge with information on how mature and well informed you are or if having the abortion is in your best interest. In most cases, interviews are scheduled for the same day as the hearing, and you will meet with the psychologist or social worker in her or his office at the courthouse. Precourt interviews usually last about 30 minutes to 1 hour, and the questions asked will be similar to the ones you will be asked in court (see **Questions You May Be Asked,** page 71). After the interview, the psychologist or social worker will go to the hearing with you and either give evidence for you or recommend to the judge that you receive a bypass.

Note: While most precourt interviews will be informal and supportive, court-appointed psychologists and social workers may sometimes seem insensitive or brusque during these meetings—especially if they usually work with teenagers who have committed violent crimes or are repeat offenders. However detached or even hostile the person you talk with may seem, keep in mind that most court-appointed psychologists and social workers are prochoice and will usually do whatever they can to make hearings less difficult and stressful for you. In particular, if any potentially negative evidence comes up in court—for example, if you've been pregnant before or just lost a job—a psychologist or social worker may help your lawyer to reframe or present this information in a more positive way (see **Preparing for Court**, page 67).

All counseling sessions and interviews required for teens going to court will be entirely confidential. In some cases, the counselors, psychologists, or social workers you meet with will not know your name—appointments will be made for Jane Doe—and records of counseling sessions, interviews, or anything a psychologist or social worker says in court will be sealed after the hearing.

KEEPING IT SECRET AND OTHER PRACTICAL DETAILS

✔ Confidentiality is a major concern for many young women going to court. Scheduling a hearing, making calls, and getting out of school without parents or teachers finding out may seem impossible, especially for teenagers who have never had to make these kinds of arrangements before.

If you feel scared or concerned about being able to keep your hearing and abortion confidential, talk with your counselor or lawyer. Clinic staff and attorneys are often particularly sensitive to a teenager's need for secrecy and may be able to offer help and suggestions on how to make sure no one finds out. Here are some of the practical details you may need to think about.

Communication

Arranging a hearing means calling clinics, lawyers, and courts. In some cases a counselor or lawyer may be able to schedule appointments for you, but in others, you will have to make all the required calls yourself. Scheduling appointments and hearings can take several calls, and teenagers who are unable to make or receive calls at home will need another number where counselors, lawyers, and court personnel can reach them or leave messages.

You may be able to make or take calls at work, or you may have a friend with a pager or private number you can use. Keep in mind that if you are calling a clinic, lawyer, or court in another city or state, the call may be long distance and the charge and phone number will show up on your employer's or friend's phone bill—or on your parents' bill if you are making the call from home. Find out if your provider has a free 800 number— many now do—or if a clinic or lawyer will accept collect calls.

If calling from home, work, or a friend's house is not possible, you may also be able to make calls from the clinic during counseling or other appointments. Similarly, if a counselor or lawyer is helping you to arrange a hearing or other appointments and needs to get in touch with you, she or he may be willing to leave a confidential or "coded" message at your home or job. For example, if a counselor leaves a message for you at work, she can simply say, "Jane called," without saying she is from the clinic or even leaving a phone number.

Excuses

Going to court usually means taking time off from school or work—and coming up with an excuse for parents, teachers, a boss, or other family members or friends. You may be uncomfortable with lying or forging notes, but if you are going to court it may be necessary. In some cases, a supportive adult, such as an older sister or teacher, may be willing to sign a note for you, or you can ask your lawyer if she or he can write you an excuse. Most providers will also give you medical excuses, but only for appointments at the clinic (see **Chapter 6**).

A written excuse—whoever signs it—may not ensure complete confidentiality. A note from a lawyer saying you are needed in court could raise suspicions at school, and a teacher or administrator could decide to call your parents to make sure you have their permission. Similarly, your parents could call the school if they see an unexplained absence on your report card, and in most cases, school administrators will show them whatever written excuses they have in your records.

You should also speak with your lawyer or counselor if you are concerned about running into someone you know at court. Amelia Adams, a prochoice lawyer in Kentucky, tells teenagers to say they are "following her around for the day" as part of an internship or school research project. If a court official you are supposed to speak with is a friend of the family, you should tell your lawyer or counselor ahead of time or specifically ask to speak with someone else when you get to court.

Transportation

In a few cases, a lawyer may agree to pick you up at school or meet you at the clinic or her office and drive you to court, but generally you will be responsible for arranging your own transportation to all appointments, interviews, and court hearings. Using public transportation may be possible if you live in or near an urban area; otherwise, you will have to rely on a boyfriend, older family member, or another supportive adult for rides to and from court and the clinic.

Note: Any adult who drives a minor to a court or clinic in another state can be prosecuted for violation of custody or other child endangerment laws, and while this is rare, such cases do occur. If you are crossing state lines for an abortion and are concerned about your driver being prosecuted, whoever you ask for a ride should be under 18.

Punctuality is important. Many counselors, lawyers, and judges view a young person's ability to get to meetings on time as a sign of her maturity, so be sure that whoever you ask for a ride is reliable and that you have clear directions to the clinic, lawyer's office, or courthouse. You should also have phone numbers for the clinic and your lawyer and call whomever you need to immediately if you are going to be late or if you change your mind at the last minute and decide not to go to court or have an abortion.

Even if you have a judicial bypass and do not have to tell your parents about the abortion, you may still need a friend or another responsible adult to come with you to the clinic. Specifically, if you are having a second-trimester procedure or your abortion is being done with extra pain medication or laminaria, you will not be allowed to leave the clinic alone and will need someone to drive you home. At some clinics, your driver will have to come with you and stay in the waiting room during your appointment; she or he will not be allowed to just drop you off and pick you up after the abortion (see **Chapter 9**).

AFTERCARE

Following your abortion, your clinic will give you special instructions on how to take care of yourself after the procedure and what to do if you are concerned about abnormal cramps, bleeding, or any other symptoms of postabortion complications (see **Chapter 9**). Following these instructions could put your confidentiality at risk, especially if you have parents or other family members who monitor your health and personal habits closely.

For example, some parents regularly monitor their daughters' periods. After your abortion, you may bleed for several days, or up to 2 weeks, and will only be able to use sanitary pads—no tampons. You may also have to take antibiotics for several days after the abortion to prevent infection—and some schools require teenagers taking any prescription drugs to have a note from their parents or a doctor.

Following all aftercare instructions is essential. If you are concerned about your parents or school finding out about your abortion, talk with the clinic about how to follow aftercare instructions without arousing suspicions. You should also keep your lawyer's phone number. Call her or him if complications do develop and you need to go to a hospital for emergency treatment. In such instances—which are extremely rare—your parents will have to be notified and your attorney may be able to answer any questions they have about the notification or consent law in your state and why you could legally have an abortion without telling them.

PREPARING FOR COURT

In most cases, before you go to court, you will receive additional counseling either from your attorney or a counselor at the clinic to help you prepare for the hearing. These precourt sessions generally include information on what the hearing will be like, what to wear, how to act in court, and what type of questions you may be asked. The details of the counseling you receive will vary depending on the judicial bypass procedures—and the judges—in your area. In some cases, court preparation will be part of the preabortion counseling you receive at the clinic. In others, your lawyer may meet with you for an hour or longer and give you detailed information on the hearing and the questions you may be asked.

How well you prepare for court can make your hearing less intimidating and stressful. What you wear and how you act in court are often seen as important indications of your maturity. Going over the questions you may have to answer during the hearing will help you appear more articulate and confident in court, whatever embarrassing or hostile questions a judge may ask (see **Antichoice Judges,** page 75).

If you meet with your attorney before the hearing, make sure you go over any potentially negative information that could come up in court—for example, if your boyfriend is married or you have been in court before for other reasons. In such cases, it is essential that you trust your lawyer. *Do not hide or lie about any information that could affect the outcome of your hearing,* no matter how embarrassing or "bad" you think it is. As long as you are completely honest about yourself and your current situation, your lawyer will be able to give you advice on how to answer any difficult or hostile questions and will usually be able to present, or reframe, potentially negative information in a more positive way.

"Any aspect of a teen's life, anything that she thinks of as negative, can be framed to show her maturity," says Julie Field, a prochoice attorney who formerly worked with teenagers in Michigan. "The fact that she doesn't want to tell her parents shows maturity because she is respecting their feelings. If she got fired from her job at the dry cleaner's, that shows maturity because now she'll have more time for schoolwork. Anything can be reinterpreted this way, and if you're going to court, that's the way you've got to think."

What to Expect at the Hearing

While many young women feel understandably nervous and frightened before a judicial bypass hearing, some have found that going to court is less traumatic than they expected. Remember, the hearing is *not* a trial. There will be no jury or prosecuting attorney, and in many cases, you will not have to sit in the witness stand or even be in a courtroom. Many judges hold judicial bypass hearings "in chambers"—which means in their own offices—or in other, smaller rooms in the courthouse. To make teens feel more comfortable and less scared, some judges will sit at a table with you, rather than behind a desk, and many do not wear their robes.

Hearings last 10 to 30 minutes, and during this time teens are usually, but not always, questioned by their lawyer or the judge. In some cases, your name may be used in court, but in others, you will be referred to only as Jane Doe or your initials will be used. A court-appointed psychologist or social worker may give evidence or recommend to the judge that you receive a bypass, and in a few instances, your boyfriend or another support person may be allowed in the room. Besides you, your lawyer, the judge, and court personnel, no one else will be in the room during the hearing, and all records of the proceedings will be kept completely confidential.

Note: While some teenagers feel more comfortable with a support person in the room, lawyers often recommend having your boyfriend, or anyone else who comes with you, wait outside until the hearing is over. Having a support person in court is sometimes seen as a sign of immaturity—a friend or teacher might try to "help" you answer questions with nods, winks, or other signals—and if a boyfriend or family member is present, he or she could be questioned by the judge as well. The only time having a family member present might be helpful, or required, is if you are having a hearing because you live in a state with a two-parent notification or consent law and only one of your parents has signed the forms. In such cases—for example, if your parents are divorced, and you and your mother have decided not to tell your father—a parent's presence in court may mean the hearing will last only a few minutes, and the judge will automatically grant the bypass (see **Chapter 3**).

In most cases, the bypass is granted at the end of the hearing. You can expect to leave court with whatever forms or legal documents you will need to have an abortion, or they will be delivered directly to the clinic. Your provider *must* have the bypass papers to perform your abortion, so if you receive the documents at court, be sure to take them with you when you go to the clinic. If the bypass is denied, your lawyer will talk with you about refiling or appealing the case (see **If the Judge Says No,** page 77).

What to Wear

Most lawyers tell young women to dress for court as if they were going to church or for a job interview. Wear a dress, skirt, or nice pair of pants. In some cases, wearing blue jeans to court may be okay, but be sure they are clean and wear a nice shirt or sweater with them. Do *not* wear ripped or tattered jeans, very short or tight skirts or dresses, tight or low-cut tops, heavy makeup, teased hairdos, or large, gaudy jewelry.

If you wear a uniform to school, talk with your counselor or lawyer about whether or not you should wear it to court. In some cases, wearing a uniform may help you make a good impression on the judge; in others, it could mean the judge or other court personnel may be able to figure out where you go to school. This could put your confidentiality at risk or lead to negative or hostile remarks—for example, "If you go to such a good school, why weren't you smart enough to use birth control." On the other hand, if your parents or other family members might get suspicious if you leave home dressed up for court, think about hiding a skirt or a nice pair of pants in a backpack or book bag—or borrowing clothes from a friend—and changing before the hearing.

Finally, cover up tattoos and remove the studs or other jewelry from multiple or nontraditional body piercings. If there's something you can't cover up or remove—for example, if you've just shaved your head or dyed your hair bright blue—don't apologize or act defensive or defiant about it. "It's better to own up to things up front," says the Reverend Velvet Rieth, director of a clinic in Louisiana. "If you have pink hair, tell the judge how proud of it you are. You might want to begin by saying, 'Yes, Your Honor, I know I have fuchsia hair, but don't let that stop you. I'm really smart, don't be fooled by my trappings.'"

How to Act

In general, your behavior in court should be respectful, attentive, and articulate. When answering questions, speak loudly and clearly enough so the judge can hear you. Say "yes" and "no," not "yeah" or "uh-uh." Be particularly respectful when speaking to the judge; call her or him "Your Honor," and make eye contact with the judge—don't look down or away—when answering questions. Pay attention to the proceedings, even if you are confused or aren't sure about what's going on. Don't chew gum, fidget, or play with your clothes, hair, or jewelry.

Answer all questions truthfully and completely, but *don't* offer any information you are not asked for. For example, if the judge asks if your boyfriend knows you are having an abortion, answer, "Yes, Your Honor," but don't say how old he is, if he's in school or working, or even if he supports your decision to terminate the pregnancy. In such instances, volunteering information could lead to additional, possibly intrusive or uncomfortable, questions and potentially negative evidence being revealed in court. At the same time, you should *never lie or try to conceal information.* If you are concerned about potentially negative information being revealed in court, talk about it with your lawyer *before* the hearing.

Being respectful and mature in court does *not* mean that you have to cover up your feelings or act completely unemotional. It is all right to express your emotions as long as you do it in an appropriate way—for example, telling the judge you are scared or nervous, or even crying a little bit if you are upset. On the other hand, avoid inappropriate or unconscious behavior such as smiling or laughing when you feel nervous or are asked an embarrassing question.

Finally, whatever a judge says to you, whatever intrusive or insensitive questions you are asked, don't get angry, apologetic, or hostile (see **Antichoice Judges,** page 75). You haven't done anything wrong and have nothing to be ashamed of. Judicial bypass hearings are the result of parental notification and consent laws that are largely unfair and unnecessary, and the fact that you are in court at all is a sign of your maturity and your ability to make, and take responsibility for, your own decisions. If you are confident and respectful—of the court and yourself—in most cases, you will get the bypass.

QUESTIONS YOU MAY BE ASKED

Going to court often means you will be asked certain personal or intrusive questions about school, work, family, and your pregnancy. Similar questions may also come up during prehearing interviews. While answering these questions may mean revealing embarrassing or potentially negative information, remember that all interviews and hearings will be confidential. In addition, once you've answered personal questions in precourt meetings, they will be less intimidating, and easier to answer, during your hearing.

At the same time, keep in mind that being well prepared for your hearing does *not* mean looking bored or smug or answering questions automatically. No matter how many times you've been asked specific questions, try not to look or sound like you've memorized the answers or are just reciting what someone else has told you to say.

The questions asked at a judicial bypass hearing generally focus on three main issues: if a young woman is mature or well informed enough to make her own decision and if having an abortion is in her best interest. Specific questions will vary from court to court, and in some cases, judges do ask inappropriate or irrelevant questions (see **Antichoice Judges,** page 75).

Are You Mature?

In most cases, your maturity will be judged by conventional middle-class standards, such as your grades or if you have a part-time job. You may also be asked some seemingly irrelevant questions like, "Who is the president of the United States?" These questions are intended to show that you are mentally competent. Here are some of the questions you can expect.

- Are you in school? How are your grades?

- Are you involved in any extracurricular activities, such as sports, student government, school clubs, or community service organizations?

- Do you have a part-time job? Have you filed an income tax return?

- Do you have responsibilities at home? Do you help with cleaning, laundry, shopping, cooking meals, or taking care of younger brothers or sisters?

- Do you have a driver's license? Do you have a car? Who paid for it?

- What are your plans for the future? Do you want to go to college? Are you taking courses to train for a particular career?

- Are you currently under the influence of drugs or alcohol?

- Have you ever hurt yourself or thought about hurting yourself?

- What important decisions have you made in your life so far? How do you make decisions?

Are You Well Informed?

The judge will also want to know if you have been informed about all your reproductive options. Questions here may include the following:

- Have you received counseling on all your options, including adoption and carrying the pregnancy to term?

- Do you understand the abortion procedure and its risks? What happens during the procedure?

- How long have you been pregnant?

- Have you talked with anyone else about your decision to have an abortion? Who? Is anyone putting pressure on you or trying to force you to have an abortion?

- Why don't you think you can tell your parents you are pregnant and want to have an abortion?

- Have you received counseling on birth control? Are you currently using birth control, or do you plan to after the abortion?

- What will you do if you start bleeding really heavily after the abortion? Who will you call? What will you tell your parents?

Is It in Your Best Interest?

Questions about a minor's "best interest" are usually asked only in special circumstances, for example, if the teenager seeking the bypass is very young, 14 or under; if the pregnancy is the result of rape or incest; or if telling her parents could put a young woman at risk for physical or emotion abuse. If you are 14 or under, a lawyer will usually try to show that if you are not mature enough to decide to have an abortion, you are also not mature enough to carry a pregnancy to term and abortion is therefore in your best interest. If a lawyer is trying to show that you could be at risk for physical or emotional abuse, questions will focus in more detail on what may happen if your parents find out you are pregnant. For example, you could be asked if your parents abuse drugs or alcohol or if they have threatened to hit you or throw you out of the house if you ever got pregnant. You or your lawyer could also be asked for documentation of past incidents of abuse, such as police reports or reports from child protection agencies.

YOU CAN DO IT!

✔ Getting a judicial bypass may feel like taking a test—or getting through an obstacle course—and in many ways it is. It requires determination and the ability to deal with the practical details of arranging a hearing and getting to court. Providers note that most teens who go to court are older, 16 or 17, or have a supportive adult, such as a teacher or older sister, to help with money, appointments, and transportation.

If you feel intimidated by going to court or concerned about how to answer particular questions, talk with your counselor or lawyer. Keep in mind also that while wearing appropriate clothes or having good grades may impress a judge and make a hearing a little less difficult and stressful, they are *not* essential. Even if your grades are only so-so or you just got fired from a job or you can only wear blue jeans to court, you can still get a judicial bypass. Everything you have to do to go to court—getting a pregnancy test, filing a petition, arranging appointments and time off from school—shows you are mature and responsible. In most cases, *if you can get to court, you will get the bypass.* Denials do occur, but not very often, and they can usually be overturned within a few days, either on appeal or by refiling (see **If The Judge Says No,** page 77).

"AT FIRST I WAS NERVOUS": JANE'S STORY

Jane was 17 and living in a state with a parental consent law when she became pregnant and decided to have an abortion. Like many teens who live in states with parental involvement laws, she found that going to court was not as scary as she expected, and she was relieved when the hearing was over.

After getting a pregnancy test and deciding she did not want to tell her parents, Jane received counseling at a local family planning center and was referred to a clinic where she was given information on how to get a judicial bypass.

> My father has very high expectations for his daughters. My older sister got pregnant when she was 17, and she's doing okay now, but he's gotten stricter and more conservative since then, and I didn't think he would understand this time. I talked about it with a counselor at the clinic, and she wrote a letter explaining my situation to the judge and told us where to go at the courthouse.

Jane and her boyfriend went to court the same day, even though she was concerned about running into a family friend who worked there. After filing some forms and waiting for about an hour, they were able to see a judge.

> At first I was nervous because we had to go to the clerk of court window and the man who is the clerk of court knows my dad. I was frantic. We talked with one of the women working there, and she told us we didn't have to see him; we would see another judge. They gave me a piece of paper that said "Special docket," and I had to go upstairs. They moved us around to all these different rooms, and at first they wouldn't let my boyfriend come in, but we finally got to see the judge.

Jane met her court-appointed lawyer at the hearing, which, she recalls, was held in a small courtroom and took about 10 minutes. She sat at a long table with microphones on it.

> The lawyer asked questions just to make sure we were intelligent people and this wasn't a rushed decision. She asked about school, what were our plans, how we would deal with it if we couldn't get an abortion. She asked our reasons for having the abortion—the basic questions a counselor would ask. As soon as she finished the questions, the judge said I was responsible and capable enough of speaking in my own behalf to have an abortion. I was so happy when I got out of there.

ANTICHOICE JUDGES

✶ While the majority of judges conduct judicial bypass hearings quickly and fairly, for some teens going to court will mean facing an antichoice judge and the insensitive or inappropriate questions she or he may ask. According to providers and lawyers, in some cases antichoice judges have kept young women in court for an hour or longer and quizzed them endlessly and in detail about their personal lives, the abortion procedure, and the gestational age of the fetus. Judges have tried to make teenagers change their minds by giving them inaccurate or misleading information about fetal development or the risks of abortion. Some judges with adopted children have even brought out their own family photos and urged young women to carry their pregnancies to term and relinquish the children for adoption.

A judge's statements in court may range from mildly condescending to blatantly untrue, and while there may be little you or your attorney can do to stop such remarks, this does *not* mean you won't get the bypass. Again, whatever a judge says during the hearing, most parental notification and consent laws state that if a minor is mature and well informed, the bypass *must* be granted.

If you get an antichoice judge, here are some of the inappropriate questions or comments you may hear:

* How long have you been having sex? How many boyfriends have you had?

* How did you get pregnant? Why weren't you using birth control?

* How are you going to feel later on if you kill your baby?

* I know this seems like a crisis you can't share with your family, but don't you think you should tell your parents? Oh, come on, don't you think your parents will be concerned and want to help you?

* Do you know you might become sterile? Would that change your mind?

* Have you thought about going ahead and having the baby? There's always adoption.

* Does the fetus have a heartbeat yet? Are you aware the fetus has eyes now?

* I hope this is a decision you will not live to regret, but I'm sure it will be.

+ What is a suction cannula?

+ Even though you don't have to wait, I wish you would think about it for another week.

What's the best way to respond? Whatever a judge says, try not to show that you are mad or upset. "Don't let the judge rattle you," says Rachael Pirner, an attorney who does judicial bypass cases in Kansas. "Maintain your eye contact with the judge. Maintain your composure."

.Pirner and other attorneys also agree that talking with your lawyer before the hearing can help you feel more prepared for an insensitive or antichoice judge. Your lawyer may know ahead of time who the judge will be and what kinds of questions and remarks you can expect. "I give them suggestions on how to react," says Amelia Adams. "I tell them to take your time. If you don't understand what a judge is asking, tell him you're not sure. If you're really thrown for a loop, take a deep breath and I'll object."

Adams adds that most young women handle themselves well in court and seem to know instinctively how to answer even the most difficult and upsetting questions. "The kids know exactly what they're doing when they get to court," she says. "I had one case where a judge said to a teen, 'Do you know there's a large segment of the population that feels what you're doing is murder?' Of course, that's an untrue statement, but the girl looked at him and said, 'Well, they don't have to have this baby, do they?'"

Keep in mind also that the way a judge acts in court may have nothing to do with you personally. Many judges do not like parental involvement laws, and they do not like doing judicial bypass hearings. Some are truly uncomfortable or have conflicting feelings about abortion, and even judges who are prochoice may be concerned that antichoice groups will say they are not being "thorough" if they do not ask certain personal or intrusive questions. In other cases, a judge who seems particularly hostile or intimidating may be just as embarrassed or uncomfortable as you are.

Jamie Sabino, a lawyer in Massachusetts, says that one of the judges who does bypass hearings in her area "is so embarrassed about the whole thing, he never looks at the young women, he always looks at papers on his desk. I was in a hearing with him once, and he asked the young woman if she knew what happened during the abortion procedure. She launched right into it. 'Yes, Your Honor. I'll come into the exam room and I'll put my feet in the stirrups and they'll dilate my cervix.' He said, 'No, no. I don't want to know. I just want to know that you know.' He got all red in the face and then gave her the bypass."

IF THE JUDGE SAYS NO

If your bypass is denied for any reason, *don't panic.* Whatever the judge says, try not to look angry or upset, and let your lawyer do the talking. Bypasses are often denied for no apparent reason—some judges simply refuse all bypass petitions. The case can be refiled or appealed, and the denial reversed or overturned, often within a few days.

If the case is **refiled,** your lawyer will resubmit the petition and you will have another hearing with a different judge in the same or another county. The second hearing will be similar to the first—the lawyer and judge will ask you questions—and in some cases, you may have to receive additional counseling before the second hearing, specifically if the bypass was denied because the judge said you were not well informed.

If your case is **appealed,** a second petition and a legal document about the case, called a **brief,** must be filed with the appeals or appellate court, which is a higher court that has the power to overturn the denial. Appeals hearings are different from judicial bypass hearings: they are more formal and usually take place in a courtroom. Your lawyer will tell you if you have to go to court for the hearing and whether or not you will have to answer any questions. In most cases, teenagers are not questioned during appeals hearings.

While refilings and appeals are usually handled as quickly as possible, arranging these hearings can mean that your abortion will be delayed for a day or two, or in some cases, up to a week or longer. In particular, appeals can take a week or more to arrange, depending on how long it takes your lawyer to file the necessary papers. Almost all denials are overturned on appeal; however, young women sometimes decide to tell a parent or go out of state rather than wait for a second hearing.

THE JUDICIAL BYPASS: AT A GLANCE

• A judicial bypass hearing is *not* a trial. If a judge finds that you are mature or well informed enough or that having an abortion is in your best interest, the bypass *must* be granted.

• Hearings must also be *quick, free, and confidential.* In most cases, you will have a court-appointed lawyer and will not have to pay any court or lawyer's fees. After the hearing, all court records about the case will be sealed.

- Bypass hearings usually last 10 to 30 minutes, and the only people in the room will be you, the judge, your lawyer, and a court clerk or court reporter. A court-appointed psychologist or social worker may also be present, and your boyfriend or another friend or family member may be allowed in the room.

- Your clinic will be able to tell you what you have to do to arrange a hearing in your area. Arranging a hearing can take a few days or up to a week, so *the sooner you call a clinic, the more time and options you will have.*

- You will probably have to miss school, and get someone to write excuses for you, so that you can go to court and other appointments with lawyers, counselors, and the clinic. Being on time is important, so have a reliable driver and call the clinic and your lawyer if you're going to be late.

- A driver over 18 years old can be prosecuted for taking you to another state for an abortion. If necessary, find someone who is under 18 to drive you to court or the clinic.

- *Tell your lawyer everything!* Don't try to hide or lie about any personal information, however embarrassing or "bad" it may be.

- Dress for court as if you were going to church or a job interview. A nice dress, skirt, or pants are best.

- Answer any questions a lawyer or judge asks you clearly and directly. Say "yes" and "no," not "yeah" or "uh-uh," and call the judge "Your Honor."

- Going to court can be scary, and some judges may ask insensitive and embarrassing questions. Remember that everything you do to arrange a hearing shows you are mature enough to make your own decisions. In most cases, *if you can get to court, you will get the bypass.*

- At the end of the hearing, the bypass will be given to you directly or delivered to the clinic. The clinic must have the bypass papers at the time of your appointment. If you get the papers at court, be sure to *take them to the clinic.*

- If the judge says no, *don't panic!* Your lawyer can refile or appeal the case. Minors who refile or appeal almost always get a bypass.

5

IF YOU

THINK

YOU CAN'T

AFFORD IT

Read this chapter if you want to have an abortion but are worried about your ability to pay or can't afford the clinic's fees right now.

For many women the biggest obstacle to getting an abortion is trying to pay for it. According to the National Network of Abortion Funds, lack of money may keep as many as one in five women in the United States from getting the abortions they want.

For some women, figuring out finances may mean asking a husband or boyfriend to pay a part of the abortion fee or even delaying an appointment a couple of weeks or months to save up enough money. For others—such as teenagers, women on welfare, and working women without health insurance—even raising a few dollars may seem impossible. These women sometimes become so desperate that they risk their lives by resorting to coat hangers, knitting needles, Drano, bleach, or potentially lethal herbal teas to induce an abortion (see **Chapter 8**).

While an unplanned pregnancy can be terrifying, especially if you can't afford an abortion, don't panic and don't try to induce your own abortion; it could kill you. Even if your situation feels hopeless, even if you don't have a cent, you can get help. You can get a medically safe, legal abortion. Finding financial assistance is not easy—it takes determination and persistence—but it can be done.

Today, many prochoice clinics and doctors are willing to work with women who can't afford an abortion. You may be able to arrange a payment plan or negotiate a reduced fee with your provider, and counselors will talk with you about how to raise the money you need as quickly as possible. Help may also be available from abortion assistance funds—a small but growing number of local and national groups that give grants and interest-free loans to women who may not be able to raise money for an abortion any other way.

This chapter contains information on what to do if you want to have an abortion but are worried about paying for it. The topics covered include:

• Why you should call a clinic and get counseling even if you think you can't afford an abortion

• Different ways you may be able to raise money or pay for your procedure

• How to find out if there is an abortion assistance fund in your area and what to expect when you call

---

CALL A CLINIC AND ASK FOR HELP *NOW!*

Providers say that women who need financial assistance often delay calling clinics because they feel uncomfortable, ashamed, or afraid about asking for help—or are trying to raise the money on their own. Others, particularly teenagers, may try to deny they are pregnant, thinking if they ignore the situation, it will "go away."

However common, and understandable, such feelings may be, women who delay contacting a clinic often find they are facing more problems, and fewer options, when they finally do call. The longer you put off calling, the more likely you will need a second-trimester abortion, which could mean you will have more money to raise and less time to raise it.

While an abortion during the first trimester—up to the 12th or 13th week of pregnancy—currently costs between $300 and $450, fees for second-trimester procedures—up to the 24th or 25th week—range from $400 to over $2,500. Only about half of all clinics perform "second tris," so finding a provider may also be more difficult and you may have to raise money for travel to another city or state (see **Chapter 6**).

Remember, just because you don't have the money for an abortion doesn't mean you can't call a clinic. Most clinics offer financial options counseling for women who are concerned about how they are going to pay for treatment. Some clinics even have their own small abortion assistance funds and may be able to give you a grant or loan (see **Abortion Assistance Funds**, p. 83).

> ### PAYMENT OPTIONS

When you call a clinic, a counselor or other staff member will talk with you about how much your abortion will cost and how you intend to pay for it. Most clinics offer several payment options—cash up front is not the only way to pay—and reduced or partial fees may also be available. Payment options will vary from clinic to clinic and, in some instances, decisions about what kind of payment a provider will accept are made on a case-by-case basis. For example, if you are 12 weeks pregnant and $50 short, some type of payment plan can usually be arranged to avoid delays and ensure that a more expensive second-trimester procedure does not become necessary.

Here are some of the payment options that may be available.

Private Health Insurance

At present, about two-thirds of all private health insurance plans pay for abortions. While many women in the United States do not have insurance, those who do often don't know, or are afraid to ask, if their plan has abortion coverage. "Women need to believe they have a right to abortion," says Sue Steketee, the director of a clinic in New Mexico. "They need to believe they have a right to information—to make phone calls and ask questions. It's really normal to call an insurance company and say, 'Will you pay for an abortion?'"

If you are covered by a partner's or parent's plan, they will receive notification of any medical treatment you receive. In most cases, notification forms will not specify that you have had an abortion. A general code for outpatient surgery or family-planning care is often used, but the doctor or clinic's name will be given.

Medicaid

Medicaid is government-funded health insurance coverage made available to certain individuals and families receiving welfare, disability, or other state or federal support for unemployed or low-income people. In most cases, if you receive welfare (formerly Aid to Families with Dependent Children and now called Temporary Assistance to Needy Families) or disability payments, you will be eligible. If you are pregnant and under 18 or unemployed, you may also be eligible.

At present, Medicaid pays for abortions in 17 states. Another 31 states allow payments in cases of rape and incest and to save the life of the mother (see **Appendix 1**). Your clinic will be able to tell you if it accepts Medicaid. Some providers don't, even in states where abortion is covered. A clinic may also be able to give you information on how and where to apply for Medicaid if you are eligible but not currently enrolled. Temporary coverage can often be arranged in a matter of days.

Note: Even if a clinic does not accept Medicaid, it may offer reduced fees for Medicaid-eligible women. Reduced fees are available at many clinics, and the average reduction is about $50. Your clinic will tell you if you qualify for a reduction and whether you will need to bring a Medicaid card or similar documentation with you at the time of your appointment.

Credit Cards

Credit cards are accepted at many clinics. While some women are concerned about the high interest rates most credit card companies charge, keep in mind that paying with plastic can mean the difference between a first- or second-trimester procedure or being able to get an abortion at all. Having a medically safe, legal abortion is worth the cost of the interest, however high. If you've got a card, or can borrow one from a friend, use it.

Partial Payments and Reduced Fees

Women sometimes delay making an appointment for an abortion because they only have part of the money and are attempting to raise the rest. If this is your situation—and especially if any delay will increase the price of your abortion—you may want to try negotiating a payment plan with your provider.

"Sometimes, women don't realize they can negotiate," says Loren Shelton, a volunteer with an abortion assistance fund on the East Coast. "If you don't have the money, you can say, 'I can't afford to pay this all at once.' Health care workers will often work with you. You don't have to be embarrassed or ashamed about not having money. Not many people keep emergency cash lying around—not many people can."

Some clinics may also be willing to reduce their fees if you have your pregnancy test and lab work done elsewhere. These tests are a standard part of any prenatal examination, so they may be covered by your insurance plan or by Medicaid, even if the abortion is not. You can have the tests done by your regular doctor or at a public health clinic and take the results to your abortion provider.

Note: The free pregnancy tests offered by crisis pregnancy centers—the phony clinics run by antichoice groups—are *not* medically reliable and will not be accepted by a licensed doctor or clinic. In most cases, phony clinics are not licensed medical facilities and cannot perform medically reliable pregnancy tests, prenatal exams, or other lab work. Even if you have a test done and receive "certification" of the results from a phony clinic, your abortion provider will require you to be retested (see **Chapter 1**).

ABORTION ASSISTANCE FUNDS

Payment options, and the availability of reduced fees, vary widely from clinic to clinic, and in some cases, a woman who cannot afford to pay for her own abortion may need more help than an individual provider can offer. In such instances, the clinic, or other people or prochoice groups, may be able to refer you to an abortion assistance fund.

In the past decade, abortion assistance funds have provided grants and interest-free loans to thousands of women facing a range of difficult—often desperate—personal and financial circumstances: pregnant teenagers afraid to tell their parents, women in abusive relationships, single mothers, both working and on welfare, students, women with a history of drug and alcohol abuse, HIV-positive women, and even women in prison. According to one fund, one-third of the women it assists have full- or part-time jobs but are still unable to raise the money they need for an abortion.

What Funds Can—and Can't—Do

While funds try to help as many women as possible, the assistance they offer is often limited. Women applying for help need to have realistic expectations about what these groups can and can't do.

Most funds pay for one abortion per woman and grants and loans cover only a part of the abortion fee—usually a quarter to a half. Women are expected to raise the rest on their own. Grants or loans for a first-trimester abortion usually range from $100 to $200, and for a second-trimester abortion, $250 to over $800. Whatever amount is given, the money is paid directly to the providers and, in most cases, can only be applied to the cost of the abortion itself. A few funds pay for travel and re-lated expenses—bus fares, hotels, or child care—but most do not.

Note: In a few states, local groups called practical support networks may be able to arrange rides and overnight housing for women traveling to clinics from other cities and states. Your clinic will know if there is a net-work in your area and will give you a referral number or other contact in-formation (see **Chapter 6**).

The majority of abortion assistance funds are restricted geographically. To qualify, you must live, or at least be going to a clinic, in the area where the fund is located. Some clinics have small, in-house funds, used primar-ily to help their own clients. Other funds have special arrangements with one or more prochoice clinics in their area, and women receiving help from the fund are automatically referred to one of these providers for their abortion.

A very small number of national funds provide help to women regard-less of where they live or where they are having their abortion. These funds are especially committed to helping women who do not qualify for other funds or need extra assistance to supplement a grant or loan they have already received. You can apply and receive assistance from more than one fund at a time. Funds often contact, or refer women to, each other in emergency situations or if they are unable to give a woman the full amount she needs.

Finding a Fund near You

While the number of abortion assistance funds has grown steadily in re-cent years, finding a fund near you can still be difficult. Not all cities and states have funds—in fact, many do not—and women in isolated or rural areas may have a particularly hard time getting information.

In addition, most funds are not listed in local Yellow Pages, so in most cases, you will need a referral from a clinic or local prochoice organiza-tion. Other groups and individuals who may know about funds in your area include:

+ Friends

+ Private doctors

- School counselors

- Social workers

- Public health clinics

- Prochoice churches

- Women's organizations, such as battered women's shelters and rape crisis centers

Information on funders is also available from the National Abortion Federation at 800-772-9100. You can call NAF Monday and Thursday, 9:30 A.M. to 1:30 P.M. and Wednesday and Friday, 9:30 A.M. to 5:30 P.M. eastern time. All calls are free and confidential. NAF refers women to members of the National Network of Abortion Funders (NNAF), a coalition of assistance funds. The line also provides clinic referrals and general information on abortion.

Note: Not all funds are members of NNAF, so just because NAF doesn't have a listing for a group in your area doesn't mean there isn't one. If you or someone you know has heard about a fund, ask your clinic or try to find another local referral.

When you call a fund for the first time, don't be surprised if you get a voice-mail message or busy signal. Many funds are run by part-time or volunteer staff who are able to answer phone calls only a few hours per day or week. Be persistent and *don't give up!* You may have to make many calls before you get through.

Interviews

By the time most women actually talk with a person at a fund, they are usually anxious and under a great deal of stress. Most funders know this and will try to make the application process as short and easy as possible.

Application procedures vary widely from fund to fund, but an interview is generally required, either on the phone or in person. During the interview, you will be asked basic personal information—your name, age, address, and phone number—how long you've been pregnant, and why you need help. Your interview could be as short as 15 minutes or last over an hour, and in some cases, detailed personal and financial information may be requested.

While some of the questions you may be asked will feel embarrassing and intrusive, interviews with funders are generally informal—there are no right or wrong answers—and the people you talk with will often be encouraging and supportive. Here are some of the questions you can expect.

* Are you working, full- or part-time, and how much do you make per week?

* Do you receive welfare, disability, or other government assistance? Do you receive food stamps?

* Do you have any kind of medical insurance, private or Medicaid?

* Do you have children? How many and how old are they?

* Are you a single parent? Do you receive any child support, and if so, how much?

* Are you under 18? If so, do your parents know about the pregnancy, and do they support your decision to have an abortion?

* What are your basic monthly living expenses—including rent, utilities, food, and transportation—for you and your children?

* When was your last menstrual period? Have you had a pregnancy test or a sonogram?

* Have you had any previous abortions? How many?

* Were you using contraception when you got pregnant? What kind?

* Have you been tested for HIV? Are you positive or negative?

* Have you used any drugs or alcohol during your pregnancy?

* Why are you choosing to have an abortion?

* Have you received counseling on all your reproductive options?

Note: According to funders, some women give inaccurate information about how long they have been pregnant because they are afraid they will not get a grant or loan if they tell the truth. Women think that if they ask for less money they will be more likely to get it, so they say they are in the first trimester when they are actually in the second or just aren't sure. *You are more likely to get the help you need if you tell the truth.* Many funds do provide assistance to women who need second-trimester abortions, and the amounts available are usually larger.

How Much Can You Raise?

During your interview, you will also be asked how much of the abortion fee you can raise on your own, and you and the funder will agree on a realistic amount. Since most funds only provide part of the fee, raising some portion will be essential, and it is seen as an important way for women to take responsibility for, and control of, their decision to have an abortion. You will be encouraged to raise as much as possible—even if it's only $50 or $25—and funders will talk with you about the different things you can do to come up with your part of the fee, for example:

• *Can you borrow from friends or family members?* If you can't borrow a lump sum from one person, funders suggest asking several people for smaller amounts. "You need to look at people as resources," says Stacey Haugland, the director of a clinic fund in Montana. "Someone you know may not agree with abortion, but they may still care about you and will support your decision. It may not be realistic to ask someone for $400, but if you can ask for $50, or $15, you're that much closer."

• *Do you have anything you can sell or any recent purchases or gifts you can return?* Funders report that women have sold, or pawned, television sets, stereos, and sewing machines to raise money for their abortions. Christmas and birthday gifts can also be returned. If you still have the receipt, you can take back any recent purchases or get cash back for items you have on lay-away plans.

• *Can you delay payments on rent or other bills?* Funders will often help women look at their monthly expenses to see if regular payments—such as rent or phone bills—can be stretched out or paid in installments. "We work with women on how to talk with their landlords about postponing rent payments or only paying a portion," says Toni Bond, an administrator with a Midwestern fund. "You can do the same thing with utility bills—pay only one-half this month."

• *Can you find work?* If you don't have a job, or even if you do, can you find some temporary or additional work? Small odd jobs, like babysitting or housecleaning, could provide the few extra dollars you need for your part of the abortion fee.

If you are unable to raise any money on your own, *don't panic!* Although most funds do have guidelines for determining who gets money and how much, they are also aware that some women are truly without resources. Funders often make decisions on a case-by-case basis and will readily break their own rules when faced with a real emergency.

Don't think you can't call a fund because you've waited too long, need too much money, don't know anyone you can borrow from, or are faced with other difficult circumstances. Funders say that they sometimes do have to make hard decisions about whom to help, but as long as they have the money, they rarely turn down a valid request for assistance. Even if you don't qualify, a fund may be able to refer you to another group that will be able to help, or staffers will talk with you about other ways to raise money.

Loan Repayment

In most cases, you will know by the end of the interview whether you are going to get a grant or a loan and how much it will be. Your funder will then call the clinic to tell them how much money is being provided and how much you will be bringing with you at the time of your appointment.

Whether you are offered a grant or a loan will depend on the individual fund; again, policies and guidelines vary widely. If you receive a grant, no repayment will be required. If you receive a loan, repayment of the full amount will be expected, and you and the funder will determine a reasonable and realistic repayment plan.

As noted, loans from assistance funds are interest-free, so you will not have to pay any extra fees or a percentage of the total. You will only have to pay the amount of the loan, and most funds are very flexible and understanding about letting women determine their own repayment schedule. Your monthly payments can be as much or as little as you think you can afford. *Be realistic*—$3 to $5 a month is okay if that's what you can do. You may also be asked to sign an agreement specifying the amount you will pay back each month, and in a few cases, you may need a cosigner—a friend or family member who signs the agreement and is responsible for making payments if you are unable to. If you are under 18, your cosigner may have to be an adult who is over 21.

Once you have started repayments, keep in touch with your funder, and call immediately if a payment is going to be late or you do not have the money to make your regular installment this month. Funds recognize that repaying loans can be difficult, especially if you are trying to pay back money you borrowed from friends or family members or are still catching up on rent or other bills. If you miss several installments, you may receive letters or phone calls from the fund, but in most cases, the fund will not sue you or try to collect the money you owe in any other way.

Your ability to pay back a loan will not affect a funder's decision to help you in the first place. Keep in mind, however, that most funds do run on tight budgets, and any money you pay back will make it possible for them to help other women who, like yourself, might not be able to pay for an abortion any other way.

YOU CAN DO IT!

Raising money for an abortion is hard work and very stressful, and according to funders, the women who are most successful at getting help are the ones who are determined and resourceful. Getting through to funds on the phone may take days, or even weeks. Some women may also feel hesitant or uncomfortable about asking friends or family members for a loan or delaying payment on rent or other bills. Again—however tired or frustrated or depressed you may feel right now—*don't give up!* In many cases, you may be surprised by the support and encouragement you receive from funders and clinic staff, and the extra efforts they are willing to make to help you piece together a payment plan or locate other financial assistance. The more determined and persistent you are, the more help you will get.

"What women are looking for in this situation is hope," says Marnie Wells, director of a national fund. "When I tell a woman, 'I believe in you, I think you can do it,' she says, 'You're right, I can do it.'"

IF YOU THINK YOU CAN'T AFFORD IT: AT A GLANCE

• *Don't try to self-abort! It could kill you!* No matter how hopeless your financial situation may seem right now, you will be able to get help— and a medically safe abortion.

• Call a clinic and get a pregnancy test as soon as possible. The longer you wait, the more money you may have to raise.

• Find out if your insurance or Medicaid pays for abortions. An estimated two-thirds of all private insurance plans pay for abortions. Medicaid-funded abortions are available in only 17 states, but many prochoice clinics offer reduced fees for Medicaid-eligible women.

- If you've got a credit card or can borrow one from a friend, use it. Paying high interest rates is better than paying for an expensive second-trimester procedure or not being able to have an abortion at all.

- See if you can negotiate with your provider. If you have part of the money, some providers may be willing to negotiate a payment plan with you. Others may be willing to discount their fee if you have your pregnancy test or lab work done elsewhere and bring the results to the clinic.

- Get creative. Borrow small amounts—$10 or $20—from several friends. Sell or pawn personal possessions, or return gifts or recently purchased items. Delay or stretch out payments on your rent, phone, or electricity bills. Baby-sit, houseclean, or work other odd jobs.

- To find out if there is an abortion assistance fund in your area, call the National Abortion Federation referral line at 800-772-9100. Referrals may also be available from clinics, friends, individual doctors, prochoice and women's groups, social workers, school counselors, public health clinics, and prochoice churches.

- *Don't give up!* Contacting a fund may take several, even dozens, of phone calls. No matter how many busy signals you get, no matter how many times you have to call back, try not to be discouraged, Keep dialing till you get through.

- Most funds require an interview either on the phone or in person. You may be asked how much you make, how long you've been pregnant, and what your current living expenses are. Don't lie about anything, however embarrassing it may seem. You are more likely to get help if you tell the truth.

- Abortion assistance funds pay only part of the abortion fee—usually a quarter to a half. All grants and loans are paid directly to the clinic. You and the funder will decide how much you are going to pay, even if it's only $50 or $25.

- If a fund gives you a loan, pay back as much as you can, even if it's only $3 or $5 per month. Any amount you repay will be used to help other women.

6

GETTING THERE

Read this chapter if you will be traveling to a clinic in another city or state for your abortion.

For many women today, traveling to a clinic in another city or state is not an option, it is a necessity. According to the Alan Guttmacher Institute, 84 percent of counties in the United States are now without abortion providers; rural areas, where one-third of women live, are particularly underserved. In certain parts of northern California, if you need a second-trimester abortion, you may be driving 5 to 7 hours; in Michigan's upper peninsula, just getting to the nearest clinic can mean 10 to 12 hours on the road.

Although the current shortage of providers has many causes—not the least of which is antichoice pressure on medical schools, hospitals, and individual doctors—the lack of a nearby clinic is not the only reason women travel. Teenagers who live in states with parental consent laws routinely go out of state, and women concerned with confidentiality may drive several hours to another city just to make sure no one they know will see them entering a clinic.

The problems associated with travel may seem simple—gas, food, a hotel room—but for many women, they can be overwhelming. What do you do if you live in a state with a 24-hour waiting period and have to take extra time off from a job with a nosy boss and no paid sick leave? How will you get to the clinic if you don't have a car, the bus to the city runs only once a day, and the nearest stop is in a town an hour away? What will you tell your coworkers, your mother, or your partner—all of whom are rabidly antichoice?

The difficulties of getting an abortion under these circumstances cannot be underestimated. It is difficult, exhausting, and extremely stressful,

91

but it is possible. Today, many providers are sensitive to the needs of women traveling long distances, and while the help they can offer is sometimes limited—for example, child care is rarely available at clinics—rules can usually be bent or stretched in emergencies. Your provider may be able to help you find a cheap hotel or schedule you for an early appointment so you can be out of the clinic in time to pick up the kids or get home before your partner. In some cases, local groups called practical support networks may also be able to help with rides or overnight housing.

This chapter contains basic information on how to plan for, and reduce, the extra time, expense, and stress of traveling to a clinic in another city or state. The material covered includes:

+ Finding the nearest clinic that has the services and scheduling options you need

+ Making a realistic travel plan, figuring out how much extra money you will need, and what clinics and practical support networks can help you with

+ Coming up with excuses for school, work, friends, and family

+ Planning for the ride home, including what to do if you experience any symptoms of postabortion complications

FINDING THE CLINIC NEAREST YOU

While time is a central concern in any decision to continue or terminate a pregnancy, for women traveling long distances to a clinic it can be critical. Arranging an abortion in another city or state can take days or even weeks, and a missed appointment can mean the difference between a first- and second-trimester procedure—and the need to find another provider, who may be located even further away. *The sooner you find a clinic and call for an appointment, the more time and options you will have for making travel plans and the less pressured you will feel.*

To find the prochoice clinic nearest you, call the National Abortion Federation or Planned Parenthood referral lines (see **Chapter 1**). The NAF referral line—at 800-772-9100—is particularly recommended for women who need a second-trimester abortion or have questions about informed consent and parental involvement laws. Referrals to abortion assistance funds are also available, and all calls are free and confidential.

Women looking for clinic referrals can also check their local Yellow Pages or call a family planning center or prochoice group in their area (see **Appendix 1**). Internet resources include the NAF and Planned Parenthood Web sites and Abortion Clinics OnLine (see **Chapter 1**).

Note: Finding a referral for a second-trimester abortion can be especially difficult for women in small towns and rural areas. Local doctors, public health nurses, or even other clinics may be unaware or misinformed about the availability of second-trimester abortions. You may even be told that the procedure is illegal. *This is not true!* You can legally terminate a pregnancy up to the 24th or 25th week—measured from the first day of your last menstrual period—and the NAF and Planned Parenthood referral lines can help you find a clinic.

Closest and Cheapest May Not Always Be Best

When faced with the current shortage of providers, women in small towns and rural areas sometimes choose a clinic just because it is the first, closest, or cheapest one they can find. Travel time and expenses are, understandably, major concerns for many women, but closest or cheapest doesn't always mean best. You don't have to make an appointment with the first clinic you call. Going to a provider you feel comfortable with—and getting the best care possible—is worth making a few extra calls, driving an extra hour, or even paying a slightly higher fee.

You should also make sure that the clinic you choose has the services you need. If you are in the second trimester, make certain you are not too far along—some clinics only go to 16 or 20 weeks—and if necessary, get a sonogram to confirm the length of your pregnancy *before* your appointment (see **Chapter 9**). If you have a physical disability or high-risk medical condition, such as asthma, let the clinic know ahead of time and ask about any special services you need (see **Chapter 1**). If you get to a clinic and find that a specific service you need is not available, you may be referred to another provider, no matter how far or long you have driven.

MAKING AN APPOINTMENT

For women traveling to a provider in another city or state, scheduling an abortion can be a fine balancing act between when the clinic performs procedures and when you can actually get there. Scheduling options and

---

IF YOU ARE UNDER 18

If you are under 18, you will need to talk with your provider about parental notification and consent laws or any other special requirements the clinic has for teens. At some clinics, women under 16 may need to have a parent or other responsible adult sign a consent form, whether or not it is legally required. You may also need an adult to come with you if you live more than 2 hours from the clinic, are having a second-trimester abortion, or are going to a provider who uses extra pain medication or laminaria for all teens (see **Chapters 3** and **9**).

Minors traveling to a clinic in another state also need to be aware of laws forbidding certain adults from transporting them across state lines or interfering with a parent's or guardian's custodial rights. In isolated cases, these laws have been used to prosecute teachers, neighbors, or other concerned adults trying to help young women get abortions. If you are concerned about your driver being prosecuted, make sure the person you ask is under 18.

---

flexibility vary widely from provider to provider and will often depend on a clinic's location—city or rural—and how many doctors it has on staff. A woman's scheduling options may also be affected by personal circumstances—such as a girlfriend who can only get off work to drive to town on Wednesdays or the need to get home before an unsupportive partner arrives.

City clinics usually have a larger pool of available doctors and are often able to schedule abortions 3 or more days a week. Some but not all will also have evening and weekend appointments. Doctor availability tends to be more limited in small towns and rural areas—one clinic in North Dakota flies in a doctor from North Carolina! In such cases, a provider may only perform abortions 1 or 2 days a week, and women may have to wait a week or longer for the first available appointment. Second-trimester or other two-day procedures may also be limited to certain days and times in a clinic's schedule. For example, a clinic may perform first-trimester abortions Tuesdays through Fridays, but see second-trimester patients only on Wednesdays and Thursdays.

In most cases, clinic staff will offer you the first appointment time they have available—not the only time. *Ask about all your scheduling options*, and don't give up if you can't find a day or time on the first call or have to reschedule one or more appointments. Most clinics will work with you to find an appointment time that meets your work and family obligations, need for confidentiality, or other personal circumstances. Extra, and at times extraordinary, efforts will also be made to see you as quickly as possible in emergency situations—for example, if waiting a week or even a few days will mean you need a more expensive procedure.

If a clinic truly does not have appointment times that meet your needs, it may be able to refer you to a nearby provider with different scheduling options. Ask about clinics you can reach by driving about the same distance, but in another direction. If the clinic 3 hours east can't see you on Saturday, the provider 4 hours south may be able to.

MAKING A TRAVEL PLAN

For some women in small towns and rural areas, long-distance travel is inconvenient, but something they do regularly. For others, just the thought of getting to a clinic in another city or state may feel overwhelming. Logistical problems—like borrowing a car, finding a place to stay, and getting time off—may seem insurmountable at first, and the social stigma of abortion and the need for confidentiality can leave a woman feeling isolated and powerless. Travel plans may have to be made quickly, in secret, or with little help from others, and essentials—such as making sure you have enough money for gas and food—may be overlooked or neglected.

To reduce the stress of getting to a clinic in another city or state, providers suggest making a travel plan. Here's one way to begin:

- *Estimate how long you have been pregnant and how much time you can wait before scheduling an appointment.* If you are currently 6 weeks pregnant, it could be easier to schedule your abortion for a month from now, when you will still be in the first trimester. If you are 11½ weeks, can you make travel plans in a few days, or will it be all right for you to wait and find a provider who performs second-trimester abortions?

Note: While waiting till the second trimester is generally not recommended, in some cases it is unavoidable. It can also give women the extra time they need to think carefully about their abortion decision and make travel or other necessary arrangements. Again, if you are uncertain about how long you have been pregnant, get a sonogram. Sonograms may be available at family planning centers, public health clinics, private doctor's offices, or hospitals; they are usually covered by private insurance plans and Medicaid. If you need a referral, ask your clinic or a local prochoice group.

- *Decide on a realistic time frame for scheduling your appointment, and work backward.* Look at a calendar or make a time line on a sheet of paper. Write down everything you will have to do to get to the clinic—borrow a car, find child care—and any help you will need to do it. Making a list may help you to feel more in control and to focus on the specific tasks that need to get done.

- *Have backup plans.* Who can you call if your boyfriend's car breaks down or your sister gets sick and can't watch the kids?

- *Don't give up!* If you miss an appointment or feel stuck or frustrated, talk with a supportive friend or call the clinic and ask to speak with a counselor. Venting or brainstorming for a few minutes may help you come up with other options or a whole different solution to the problem.

Keep in mind that the details of any woman's travel plan will depend on a range of factors, such as length of pregnancy, how far she needs to travel, and support from family and friends. Here are some of the things you may need to think about.

Transportation

For most women today, getting to a clinic means having a car or knowing someone who does. Taking a bus, train, or plane may be expensive, and even where available, service to and from rural areas and small towns is often limited or irregular and may require additional time and travel arrangements. Catching a bus or train to the city may mean a trip to the next town or a highway junction an hour away. If you have a 9 A.M. appointment, you could end up on a "red eye" that arrives in town at 3 A.M.

If you need to borrow a car or ask someone to drive you, make sure the person you ask, and their vehicle, are reliable. If you are having a second-trimester procedure or are going to use extra medication—Valium, IV sedation, or a general anesthetic—you will *not* be allowed to drive home, or even ride on a bus, by yourself. Women receiving extra pain medication may also need to have a friend or family member stay with them for at least 12 hours after the procedure to ensure they have transportation back to the clinic or to a hospital in case any complications develop.

Estimating Travel Time   Cramming an abortion and two long car trips into a single day is not only extremely stressful; it may be medically risky. Abortion is a surgical procedure, and stress may affect the amount of pain and discomfort you experience during the abortion and the likelihood of complications afterward. Be realistic about the amount of time you will need—for travel, the appointment, and recovery—and give yourself some leeway for road and weather conditions, unexpected delays at the clinic, and getting lost in city traffic.

If a 9 A.M. appointment means getting up at 4 or 5 A.M. and driving 3 or more hours, consider getting to the city the afternoon or evening before. You will have time to find the clinic and get a good night's sleep, and you will be more relaxed and focused for your abortion. You may also be able to arrange an afternoon or evening appointment for your preabortion medical tests and counseling so you won't have to spend as much time at the clinic the following day and will be able to start home even earlier.

Directions   Most clinics will give you directions when you make your appointment. *Write them down*—even if you think you know where the clinic is located—and invest in a good road or street map. In some cases, your provider may also be able to mail directions and a map to you ahead of time. If you don't want to receive mail from the clinic at home, have the information sent to you at work or a friend's address.

Even with directions, driving on unfamiliar highways or in city traffic can be intimidating or confusing, and being late for an appointment can cause additional delays or, in rare cases, rescheduled appointments. If you do get lost or are going to be late, *call the clinic immediately.* Some clinics have a special inside line or other emergency number for you to call, and you should be sure to take it with you.

What You'll Need to Take with You: A Checklist   Your clinic will also give you instructions on what to bring with you at the time of your appointment (see **Chapter 9**). Make sure you have all the required items before you leave home. In particular, security and payment policies at some clinics are strictly enforced, and a forgotten ID or credit card could mean a rescheduled appointment. Packing snacks, water, or anything else you would normally take on a long-distance car trip or bus ride will also help you to relax while you're on the road. Here's what you will need to bring.

- A picture ID or other **proof of identity.** An ID may also be required for your partner, parents, or anyone else coming with you to the clinic. In states with parental notification or consent laws, divorced or single parents may also need to bring documents showing proof of custody (see **Chapter 3**).

- The full amount of the **abortion fee** or the appropriate insurance or Medicaid forms. Credit cards are accepted at many clinics; personal checks are not.

- Extrathick **sanitary pads.** Moderate to heavy bleeding after an abortion is normal, so you may need a few pads in the car for the ride home (see **Aftercare on the Road,** p. 103).

- **Creature comforts.** Do whatever you'd normally do to reduce stress during a long drive. Wear comfortable clothes and shoes; bring along some of your favorite tapes or CDs; plan regular rest stops. If you are bringing your children, pack snacks and a favorite toy or game to keep them occupied.

Housing

Overnight housing may be necessary if you live in a state with a 24-hour waiting period, you are having a 2- or 3-day procedure, or driving to and from the clinic in one day would be too stressful or medically risky (see **Estimating Travel Time,** p. 97). At a few clinics, fees for second-trimester abortions or other 2-day procedures include an overnight hotel room, but in most cases you will be expected to arrange your own housing. Providers can usually refer you to safe, reasonably priced hotels in their area, and you can expect to pay between $30 and $60 a night.

Note: If your abortion is being performed with laminaria—generally a 2-day procedure—you may have to stay within 30 minutes to an hour of the clinic between appointments and have direct access to a private telephone. In some cases, laminaria insertion can cause moderate to heavy cramping, and these extra precautions may be necessary to ensure you can call and return to the clinic immediately if complications occur (see **Chapter 9**).

Do not sleep in your car, even in emergencies. If you are unable to arrange housing for any reason, tell the clinic ahead of time. A referral to a practical support network may be available (see **Practical Support Networks,** p. 100), or the clinic may be able to help with alternative arrangements.

Child Care

Most clinics do not provide child care and will strongly discourage you from bringing your children to the clinic. What happens if you show up with the kids in tow? At some clinics, a staff member might agree to watch the children for you, especially if they are older and can read or play quietly. At others, you will be asked to reschedule your appointment for a time when you can arrange child care.

Referrals to local child care providers are available at some, but not all, clinics. If the kids have to come with you, your best bet is to bring a partner, friend, or family member who can take care of them during your appointment. Clinic staff will often be able to give you information on local movie theaters, playgrounds, museums, or malls where the children and caretaker can go for a few hours.

Food

Don't forget to include food in your travel expenses. Some women omit meals when figuring out how much money they'll need, especially since many clinics tell women not to eat or drink for several hours before an abortion. Plan on having a good meal after the procedure—you'll need it. Food will also be essential if you are driving home alone and have not eaten since the night before. Again, most providers will be able to refer you to reasonably priced restaurants in their area.

Money

When estimating travel expenses, be realistic and don't skimp on the essentials, like gas, food, and a safe, comfortable place to stay. If a round-trip bus ticket or overnight stay is necessary, you will probably need about $100 to $200 over and above the abortion fee.

If raising money for travel expenses could delay your abortion—and especially if a missed appointment could mean a more expensive procedure—talk with the clinic about how much money you have and what you will need to cover your abortion and travel expenses. A counselor may be able to give you a few ideas on how to borrow or raise extra money, or you could get referrals to practical support networks or abortion assistance funds (see **Chapter 5**).

Keep in mind that financial assistance for travel expenses is rarely available. If you are $25 short for either the abortion fee or a bus ticket, buy the bus ticket; then talk with the clinic about arranging a grant, loan, or payment plan for the abortion fee.

IF YOU NEED PREABORTION COUNSELING

The need to make travel plans quickly and in secret sometimes complicates or becomes confused with a woman's decision to continue or terminate an unplanned pregnancy. In such instances, a woman may "numb out" or think she doesn't have time to consider all her options, and she

---

PRACTICAL SUPPORT NETWORKS

As the number of providers has steadily dwindled and women have had to travel longer and longer distances to get to clinics, concerned women and men in some communities have responded to the situation by forming practical support networks. These groups try to make sure women arriving in town for an abortion have a place to stay and rides to and from the clinic. Depending on the group, rides from other cities or towns may also be arranged, or in emergency situations, a network might provide child care or pay for a bus ticket or hotel room.

At present, the help available from practical support networks is limited. Groups exist in only a few states; they run on small budgets and may be difficult to contact. Prochoice groups and providers usually know if a network has been formed in their area and will refer women who need help. Groups may be listed in Yellow Page directories under the heading for Abortion Services, or you can try calling the NAF referral line.

In emergency situations, individual clinics may also offer women help with transportation and housing on a case-by-case basis. At one clinic in Colorado, staffers sometimes drop by the bus station to pick up women arriving in town for early-morning appointments. At others, if a woman doesn't have enough money for food or a hotel room, a small reduction in her abortion fee may be arranged. Keep in mind that individual clinics have very different guidelines about what constitutes an "emergency." The assistance they can provide in such cases is frequently limited and should not be expected or taken for granted.

may arrive at a clinic feeling angry, sad, or still ambivalent about her decision.

Women looking for preabortion counseling in rural or small-town areas need to be particularly wary of phony clinics run by antichoice groups. These so-called clinics or crisis pregnancy centers often advertise free pregnancy tests and "options" or "preabortion" counseling, but they are generally not licensed medical facilities and will not give you accurate, unbiased information on all your reproductive options (see **Chapter 1**).

If you are uncertain about your decision for any reason, speak with your provider or a local prochoice group about where to get preabortion counseling in your area. Nondirective, nonjudgmental counseling may be available from a local family planning center or prochoice clergy. Where local counseling is not available, the clinic may be able to arrange for you to speak with a counselor on the phone (see **Chapter 8**). If you arrive at a clinic and tell a counselor you are not sure about your decision or appear upset or ambivalent, your abortion may be delayed or rescheduled, no matter how many hours you have driven or how difficult it was to arrange child care or time off.

EXCUSES

If you are traveling a long distance to get an abortion—and even if you're not—getting help and protecting your confidentiality may make lying, or simply stretching the truth a little, an occasional, if uncomfortable necessity. You may need excuses at work or school, or for friends or family members who want to know why you need a ride to the bus station or someone to watch the kids.

If you aren't sure who to ask for help or need a plausible excuse for a specific person or situation, call your clinic and ask to speak with a counselor. Most clinics will not encourage you to lie outright, but they will brainstorm with you about what a partner, parent, or employer might or might not believe, how they might react if you tell them the truth, and what you feel comfortable saying to them. Here are some of the excuses that have worked well for other women.

• *Shopping.* This is one of the most commonly used reasons women give for day trips to the city and, apparently, the one least likely to raise the suspicions of friends or family members. Occasional shopping trips to larger towns or cities are not unusual for women who live in small towns and rural areas, and some women do combine abortion appointments with shopping or other personal business.

- *School or work project.* Say you have to do research at a special library, are conducting interviews, or have a special internship, seminar, or meeting.

- *Visiting or helping a friend or family member.* This is a good one to combine with a shopping trip if you have to leave home unusually early to get to the clinic: "A friend of Joan's just moved to the city, and she wants us to meet her for breakfast." "John's aunt isn't feeling well, and we said we'd drop by and run some errands for her."

- *Doctor's appointment.* In most cases, schools and employers will not question you if you say you have a doctor's appointment or are having outpatient surgery, and your clinic will provide you with a written excuse signed by a doctor. Clinics often use generic excuses stating that you have had minor surgery and should not engage in heavy physical activity for a few days. Excuses are usually written or printed on special forms or stationery that do not contain the clinic's name, address, phone number, or any other identifying information.

Note: If a teacher, school counselor, coworker, or supervisor starts asking questions about your "surgery" or why you need time off, try telling them you're being treated for "female problems." Most men, and some women, are squeamish about any mention of women's reproductive health—they think you're going to talk about menstruation—and will usually change or drop the subject quickly.

TAKING CARE OF YOURSELF

Despite the best efforts of clinics and other prochoice groups, getting to a clinic in another city or state can still be an arduous and exhausting ordeal. Women do drive all night, on bad roads, in bad weather, by themselves or with kids in the car. They arrive at clinics bleary-eyed and hungry, only to face a line of antichoice picketers, or they discover they are 2 weeks' farther along than they thought and will have to go to another provider and come up with $200 or $500 more to pay for a later procedure.

Getting an abortion under such circumstances not only takes enormous strength and determination; it is also extremely stressful. By the time some women arrive for their appointments, they are angry, upset, or hostile, and they may express or act out these feelings in inappropriate ways—for example, by yelling at counselors or being uncooperative.

Misdirected anger and other acting-out behavior are often understand-able, but they may make your appointment more difficult. Uncooperative behavior can also delay your abortion and add hours—in the waiting room, in recovery, and on the road—to an already long day.

If you arrive at a clinic feeling upset for any reason, ask to speak with a counselor. Venting or just complaining for a few minutes may help you to calm down and focus on the things you need to do to ensure that your abortion is completed as safely and quickly as possible.

AFTERCARE ON THE ROAD

While abortion is an extremely safe procedure and the likelihood of complications is less than 1 percent, clinics often take special precautions with women facing a long drive home. After the procedure, you will be given written aftercare instructions, and a nurse or counselor will go over them with you. You will also be given a 24-hour emergency number to call in case any complications occur. Make sure you have the number with you before you get back on the road (see **Chapter 9**).

If you are at all concerned about complications, think about staying in town after the procedure. If you have had a second-trimester abortion or received additional pain medication or a sedative, you will not be allowed to drive home by yourself and may need someone to stay with you for 12 hours after the procedure.

If you do not have someone to drive you home, you may have to stay at the clinic for 2 to 4 hours to ensure that the pain medication or sedative has worn off and no abnormal cramping or bleeding has occurred. You may also have to sign a medical release stating you are driving home alone against the clinic's advice. Even if you do have a driver, some providers will suggest that you stay near the clinic for 1 or 2 hours after the procedure—have a meal, go shopping, or see a movie—and then check back with them before getting on the road.

If you do need to get home immediately, here are a few extra precau-tions that will ensure that potential complications are identified and treated as quickly as possible.

- *Plan a rest stop every 1½ to 2 hours.* Regular stops are necessary so you can check your sanitary pad for abnormal clots or bleeding.

- *Walk and stretch.* During rest stops, get out of the car and do some stretching exercises or walk around for a few minutes. A little bit of ex-ercise is essential to ensure that blood does not pool or clot in your legs. If you are on a particularly long stretch of road and can't stop, keep your feet and legs moving with stretching or "pumping" exercises. Pump or treadle your legs as if you were playing an organ or working on an old-fashioned sewing machine with foot pedals.

• *Stay on major highways if possible.* In the event of an emergency, you will be able to get to a phone or hospital or return to the clinic as quickly as possible.

• *Call the clinic if you have a fever or excessive bleeding.* If your fever goes over 100.4 degrees or you are bleeding through more than one extrathick pad an hour for more than 2 or 3 hours, phone the clinic immediately. Do not go to a private doctor or hospital emergency room until you have spoken with the clinic. Treatment of complications is free at most clinics, and the quality of care is often better.

Medical personnel in small towns and rural areas sometimes have limited experience treating postabortion complications, and doctors and nurses may make insensitive remarks about your abortion or perform unnecessary surgery. For example, at many hospitals heavy bleeding is treated with an emergency D & C, a procedure that can cost between $500 and $1,000.

If your clinic does instruct you to go to an emergency room, a nurse practitioner or counselor will tell you what to say to the hospital's medical staff to ensure that you receive appropriate care. In some cases, the clinic may be able to call ahead to let the hospital know you are coming and discuss the best plan of treatment.

Follow-up Appointments

Most clinics recommend that you have a follow-up appointment 2 to 3 weeks after an abortion to make sure you have fully recovered from the procedure. If you have your follow-up appointment at the clinic, it will be included in your abortion fee. The exam should not be skipped, even if you have experienced no signs of complications (see **Chapter 9**).

If returning to the clinic for a follow-up exam means another long drive, ask for a referral to a prochoice doctor or family planning center in your area. In most cases, you will also be given a letter or medical form to take to the appointment. The letter will state that you have had an abortion and include any other information the doctor or clinic may need to do a thorough exam. If you go to a local doctor or clinic you will usually be charged for the appointment. All records of the exam will be kept confidential.

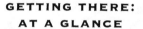

GETTING THERE:
AT A GLANCE

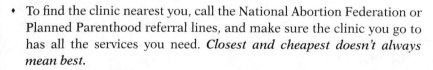

- To find the clinic nearest you, call the National Abortion Federation or Planned Parenthood referral lines, and make sure the clinic you go to has all the services you need. *Closest and cheapest doesn't always mean best.*

- If you are uncertain about your decision to terminate or continue a pregnancy, find out about preabortion counseling in your area. If you arrive at the clinic feeling ambivalent or undecided, your abortion could be delayed or rescheduled.

- To make a travel plan, figure out how long you've been pregnant and how long you can wait to schedule an abortion, then work backward. Make a list of everything you'll need to do to get to the clinic—arrange transportation, housing, child care—and who can help you.

- *Don't give up* if the first clinic you call can't find an appointment time that works for you. Not all clinics have evening or weekend appointments, so you'll probably have to take one or more days off from work or school.

- When estimating travel expenses, be realistic and don't skimp on essentials, like gas, food, and a decent hotel room. If a round-trip bus fare or overnight stay is involved, expenses of $100 to $200 can be expected.

- *Don't sleep in your car.* Your clinic can refer you to a safe, reasonably priced hotel or help you find emergency overnight housing.

- If possible, arrange for child care at home. If you have to bring the children, ask a partner, friend, or family member to come with you and look after the kids during your appointment.

- If you need an excuse for a day trip to the city, tell people you are going shopping, doing research for a school or work project, or visiting a friend or family member. If you need time off from work or school, most clinics will provide you with a written medical excuse.

- Make a checklist of everything you need to take with you—directions, ID, money—and give yourself plenty of time to get to the clinic. Be sure you have the clinic's number, and *call if you're going to be late.*

- If you feel upset when you reach the clinic, ask to speak with a counselor. Don't get mad at clinic staff. Misdirected anger or other uncooperative behavior can add stress and additional delays to your appointment.

• Make sure you have written aftercare instructions and the provider's 24-hour emergency number before you leave the clinic. If you develop a high fever or are bleeding through more than one pad per hour, *call the clinic immediately.*

• A follow-up appointment 2 to 3 weeks after the procedure is essential to make sure you have fully recovered from your abortion. If you are unable to return to the clinic for a follow-up exam, ask for a referral to a prochoice doctor or family planning center in your area.

⑦

CLINIC

HARASSMENT

Read this chapter if you are going to a clinic where antichoice picketing or harassment may be expected.

At many clinics today, antichoice picketing and harassment are an unfortunate and unavoidable fact of life. On weekends, and even weekdays, women arriving at clinics may have to cross lines of screaming, taunting protesters or face so-called sidewalk counselors who may try to talk them out of having an abortion. Blockades, firebombings, vandalism, and shootings also continue to occur, though with less frequency than in the 1980s and early 1990s.

Clinic harassment can be upsetting, frightening, or just a plain nuisance, and providers and other prochoice groups have fought back by pushing for state and local clinic access laws that make it illegal to block clinic entrances or harass patients and staff. A federal law, the Freedom of Access to Clinic Entrances (FACE) Act, was passed in 1994 (see **Clinic Access and "Bubble" Laws,** p. 116). Providers have also sued antichoice groups and individuals, spent thousands of dollars to improve security, and worked with volunteer client escort groups to ensure women can enter and leave clinic buildings as safely and quickly as possible.

Given the persistence and fanaticism of some antichoice groups, clinic harassment seems likely to continue. Certainly, antichoice groups and individuals have a constitutional right to express their opinions freely and openly. They do *not* have the right to stop women from entering clinics, to intimidate or threaten clinic patients and staff, or to try to close down licensed medical facilities. Your right to unobstructed access to a clinic and any medical treatment you choose is equally important and protected under the law.

This chapter contains basic information on what to expect if you are going to a clinic where antichoice picketing or harassment may occur. The topics covered include:

• The different ways antichoice groups and individuals may try to threaten or intimidate you

• How women feel about harassment and how to take care of yourself physically and emotionally if you are harassed

• Recently enacted federal and local clinic access laws and what clinics are doing to reduce harassment and help women get inside safely

• What you can do to avoid or reduce your exposure to picketers

ANTICHOICE HARASSMENT: WHAT TO EXPECT

Antichoice harassment varies widely from state to state and clinic to clinic. Every group of protesters seems to have their own particular tricks and methods, and how abusive and violent they get often depends on whether existing antiharassment laws and court rulings are being enforced. In some instances, enforcement is decidedly lax, and antichoice groups are constantly testing the laws or coming up with new ways to get around them.

Based on women's experiences in recent years, here are the most common types of harassment you are likely to encounter.

Prayer Vigils

Prayer vigils are often organized by religious groups, such as local churches, rather than political antichoice organizations. During a vigil, the group will stand, kneel, or walk back and forth in front of a clinic, reciting prayers or singing hymns. For example, Catholic groups who stage vigils usually recite the rosary.

While generally not illegal, prayer vigils can vary in intensity and intrusiveness. In some cases, vigil participants do not try to talk to women or prevent them from entering a clinic; they simply sing, pray, and leave. In others, they may shout or use bullhorns to amplify prayers or hymns and engage in more confrontational activities, like picketing and sidewalk counseling.

Picketing

Picketing at clinics can also vary from one or two individuals carrying signs that say "Don't kill your baby" to groups of 20 to 50 protesters who taunt and yell at women and try to give them antiabortion materials. Picketers may also try to stop you when you are driving into the clinic's parking lot, or they may try to talk or give literature to your partner or anyone else accompanying you.

Often aggressive and intensely abusive, this kind of harassment is intended to make women feel guilty or ashamed or to scare them with inaccurate or distorted information about abortion and abortion providers. Picketers frequently carry signs with pictures of stillborn or dismembered babies—in many cases, the pictures are *not* aborted fetuses, as the antichoice people claim—or they may hold up dolls or plastic replicas of fetuses. Women crossing picket lines can also expect to see a range of antichoice signs and hear slogans such as:

* Abortion is murder.

* Baby killer!

* This clinic hurts women.

* Abortion is violence against women.

* Abortion hurts!

* Women come out of here unconscious.

* We can help you get a real doctor.

* We'll give you clothes, any help you need.

* I'll give you $10,000 for your baby.

* The doctor doesn't have a license to practice medicine.

* The doctor has thousands of malpractice suits.

* Abortion is a mistake that you'll have to live with for the rest of your life.

* Abortion causes breast cancer.

* You'll never have children—you'll be sterile.

Anyone entering the clinic with you may also be harassed, and in some cases, picketers' slogans may be specifically targeted at a woman's partner, parents, or other family members; for example:

- Real men don't let their girlfriends and wives have abortions.

- You're already a parent. You're supposed to protect babies, not kill them.

- Don't let your sister become a murderer.

Sidewalk "Counseling"

So-called sidewalk counselors are in fact picketers—sometimes specially trained by antichoice groups—who approach individual women outside clinics and try to give them antichoice literature and talk them out of having an abortion. Typically, a counselor will approach a woman and try to start a conversation by saying something like, "Hi, are you going to the clinic today? Here's some literature we'd like you to have." The pamphlets are filled with inaccurate and distorted information, such as entirely false claims that an 11-week-old fetus can feel pain or that almost half of all women who have abortions will miscarry during subsequent pregnancies.

The deceptive nature of sidewalk counseling makes it particularly upsetting for some women, and it's easy to be caught off guard. Some of these phony counselors will be excessively nice, calling you "honey" and promising financial assistance and other help if you will go with them to a crisis pregnancy center (see **Chapter 1**). Others start out friendly, but turn aggressive and threatening, especially if a woman won't take their literature or talk with them. In such cases, the person who was earnestly offering "help" just a moment ago may suddenly start yelling antichoice slogans or push a plastic fetus into your hand.

Blockades

In the past, blockades usually involved large numbers of antichoice picketers—hundreds at times—who would try to close down a clinic by blocking all entrances: front and back doors, driveways, and parking lots. Women trying to enter the clinic would be stopped and surrounded or prevented from getting out of their cars. In extreme cases, picketers would lie down in front of women's cars or jump on their hoods and try to cover their windshields.

More recently, the number of picketers has decreased, and antichoice groups have staged what are called "lock-and-blocks." Protesters chain themselves to a clinic's front door or to old cars or steel drums, blocking the entrance to the parking lot. How quickly protesters are removed depends on how quickly local police respond. Even when police respond promptly, sawing through locks, towing away cars, and arresting protesters can take several hours or longer.

Under FACE, the federal clinic access law, all attempts to blockade clinics are now illegal. Antichoice groups have contested the law in court—in most cases, unsuccessfully—and continue to defy it from time to time by organizing isolated, symbolic blockades. These blockades have occasionally succeeded in closing a clinic temporarily, but no woman has been prevented from having an abortion. When a clinic is forced to close for a few hours, abortion appointments are rescheduled—if possible, for later the same day—or the provider arranges for its patients to be seen at another clinic.

Invasion of Privacy

At some clinics, antichoice groups and individuals have been able to find out, and publicize, the names of women who are scheduled for abortions on a particular day. Picketers photograph or videotape women entering clinics, or they copy down their license plate numbers and get their names, addresses, and phone numbers from a local office of the Department of Motor Vehicles (DMV). Personal information on clinic patients may also be obtained from antichoice sympathizers who work in local police or sheriff's offices.

The impact of this kind of harassment can be devastating. A woman arriving at a clinic may suddenly see a picketer holding a sign with her name on it: "Jane Smith, don't kill your baby." She may receive harassing letters or phone calls, or her partner, parents, or employer may be informed she has had, or is planning to have, an abortion even though she has chosen not to tell them. In a few cases, women's homes have been picketed.

A federal law passed in 1994 makes it illegal for state DMVs to release personal information on any individual. Predictably, antichoice groups are finding ways to circumvent the law—in one case, information on clinic patients was leaked by a government employee—and this form of harassment, while less frequent, continues to occur.

Butyric Acid Attacks

Sometimes called "liquid rescue" or "stink bombs," butyric acid is a foul-smelling, toxic chemical that is used to vandalize clinics and temporarily close them down. In a typical "acid attack" or "gassing," antichoice groups or individuals break into a clinic after hours and pour the chemical on the floor. Even if only a small amount is used, the fumes penetrate the entire clinic and, according to one staffer, smell like "56 people vomited on every surface you have."

Cleaning up after an attack is costly and time-consuming. Furniture, floors, walls, and ceilings may have to be replaced, and the smell can linger for weeks. Breathing the fumes can also cause uncomfortable but temporary side effects, such as throat and eye irritation, dizziness, and nausea. If you have an appointment at a clinic that has recently been gassed, your appointment may be rescheduled or you may be referred to another provider.

Vandalism, Arson, Shootings

In their increasingly desperate attempts to close down clinics, some antichoice groups have turned to extreme and lethal forms of violence. Glue has been poured in door locks, making it temporarily impossible for staff or patients to enter a clinic. Clinics have been firebombed and, in some cases, burnt to the ground. One clinic in northern California has been bombed three times.

Shootings have also occurred. In the past five years, two doctors, two receptionists, and one client escort have been killed. Others, including patients, have been wounded. While some, but not all, antichoice groups have publicly disassociated themselves from the individuals who have committed these crimes, many continue to believe that any form of violence is justified to prevent women from having legal abortions.

YELLING BACK: KIM'S STORY

Kim's experience at a Midwest clinic is typical of what crossing a picket line can be like. Kim was in her senior year in college when she became pregnant and decided to have an abortion. The clinic she chose was a regular target of antichoice groups, so she had been told to expect picketers and to try to ignore them.

Arriving at the clinic with her boyfriend, Kim was approached by several picketers almost as soon as she got out of her car. "They were nice at first," said Kim. "They were trying to give us brochures. They said, 'Hi, let me give you this. We want you to have this.' I looked down and saw what it was and said, 'No, you can keep it because it's not going to do any good. I don't want it.' I refused to take it, but they tried to push it into my hands. When I dropped it, they picked it up and tried to give it to my boyfriend. They were relentless."

The verbal harassment intensified when Kim's boyfriend finally took one of the brochures and jokingly told the picketers he intended to recycle it. "That did it. They started saying things like, 'Oh, you don't want to kill a tree, but you're willing to kill a baby. You want to save plants and animals and endangered species, but you'll murder your baby.'"

Following the advice they had received from the clinic, Kim and her boyfriend ignored the picketers and continued to walk toward the building. Before reaching the front door, they were stopped by a larger group of antichoice protesters, and the harassment grew worse.

"There was one man in particular," said Kim. "He took out a plastic fetus and literally pushed it in my face. He was shouting 'Look at this! Look at this! What are you doing killing your baby. You're a murderer. You don't want to do this. You don't want to kill your baby.' I got really furious. I felt so angry, I couldn't contain myself any more and started yelling back at him. I yelled, 'You have no right telling me what to do with my life. You have no idea what my situation is, what kind of circumstances I'm in right now or what would happen if I had a baby. I know why I'm here and I'm glad I'm here and you're not going to change my mind.' I was hoping this would shut him up, but it made him even madder. He started screaming back at me."

Although the picketers followed them right up to the doorway, Kim and her boyfriend were able to enter the clinic safely. The staff was very supportive, and she talked with a counselor about the harassment. After her abortion, Kim agreed to testify in court to help the clinic get an injunction against the picketers.

HOW WOMEN FEEL ABOUT HARASSMENT

Women's reactions to picketing and other forms of clinic harassment vary widely. For some, picketers are little more than a momentary, if unpleasant nuisance. For others, crossing a picket line can be devastating. Anger and frustration are also common reactions. Like Kim, many women are outraged by picketers' lack of compassion and respect for the hard choices women make about unplanned pregnancies.

Arriving at a clinic that's being picketed can also be intimidating and confusing. Even if a clinic has warned you about protesters, you may be surprised by the intensity of their efforts to change your mind or prevent you from entering the building.

Jean was married and in her thirties when she had an abortion at a clinic in the South. Surrounded by picketers before she could even get out of her car, she recalls, "I was told on the phone that there would be protesters, but I was just incredulous and actually a little bit shocked. You see this stuff happening on TV in other cities, but I had no idea it was going on here. I lived less than a mile from the clinic, and I had no inkling of what it would be like."

Providers say that women who have gone through picket lines occasionally decide to delay their abortions or seek extra counseling. However, these women almost always reschedule their appointments a day or week later. Diane Derzis, former director of a clinic in Alabama, recalls a typical case: "One time the picketers stopped a woman outside the clinic. They had her surrounded and down on her knees praying. She left the clinic that day, but a week later, she came back. She made an early-morning appointment so she didn't have to see any picketers, and she had her abortion."

However angry, frightened, or exasperated picketers make you feel, try not to let them see you're upset: That's what they want. Antichoice groups often train their members to target women who look vulnerable. If picketers see that you're hunched over, shaking, or about to cry, they may yell louder, use more abusive and threatening language, or try to hold you back or surround you so you can't get to the clinic door. According to providers, the best way to deal with antichoice protesters is to ignore them. The less you interact with picketers in any way, the less chance they'll have to harass or upset you (see **Getting in Safely: What You Can Do,** p. 117).

Note: Providers also note that a woman's partner or parents are often just as likely to be upset by picketers and yell back or try to argue with them. A violent or angry boyfriend or mother may not be able to give you the support you need, and worrying about them or trying to calm them down could make your appointment more stressful. If you think a particular friend or family member will be upset by protesters, leave them at home and ask someone else to come with you.

Women who are upset by picketers sometimes act out their feelings in inappropriate ways. Once inside the clinic, they may be rude, uncooperative, or hostile.

Given the severity of harassment some women experience, this kind of misdirected anger is understandable, but it can also be counterproductive. Refusing to cooperate with clinic staff can make your appointment longer, and any added stress during an abortion may increase your risk for complications (see **Chapter 9**).

If you are harassed by picketers and feel upset, *ask to speak with a counselor.* Expressing your emotions, even for a few minutes, may help you vent negative feelings and relax. Keep in mind, also, that most providers are already doing everything they can to stop harassment. Their efforts have played a major role in the current decrease in blockades and picketing throughout the country.

WHAT CLINICS ARE DOING

Faced with continuing antichoice harassment and violence, many clinics have instituted tight security procedures to ensure the safety of their buildings, staff, and patients. While some clinics now look more like armed camps than medical facilities, the increased security usually adds to women's feelings of safety and support. Security measures vary widely from provider to provider, and your clinic will be able to tell you about the policies and procedures it currently has in force.

Clinic Security

In the past few years, physical security has become a top priority at many clinics. Parking lots and front entranceways have been walled or fenced in—in some cases, with barbed wire. Clinics have also installed security systems that require patients to go through several locked doors and waiting areas monitored by video surveillance cameras—both outside and inside the clinic. You or anyone coming with you to the clinic may have to show a picture ID. In addition, clinic shootings have prompted some providers to install metal detectors and to inspect the contents of women's purses. Others may tell you not to bring large bags or purses to the clinic.

A growing number of clinics are also hiring private security guards. These individuals may be off-duty police officers with the authority to arrest picketers who break local trespassing or clinic access laws. At some clinics, guards may be on duty only if picketing is expected or occurring; at others, they are there whenever the clinic is open.

Note: Heavy security does not always mean a clinic is expecting or has recently experienced intensive picketing or other harassment. Specific security measures, like having a guard on duty, are often intended to reassure clinic staff or other individuals who enter and leave the building on a daily basis.

Client Escorts

Often organized by local prochoice or women's organizations—as well as individual providers—client escorts are volunteers, women and men, who stand outside clinics when a blockade or picketing is expected and help patients and staff get inside the building safely. Escorts usually wear brightly colored clothing—for example, an orange vest or T-shirt with the word *Prochoice* on it—or they may carry prochoice signs. When they come up to you, they will say something to let you know they are pro-choice volunteers, not picketers, such as "We're with the clinic. Do you need help?"

The number of escorts you can expect to see and what they will do to help you usually depends on the intensity of picketing or other harass-ment. In cases of light or moderate picketing, only a few escorts may be in front of the clinic. One or two will come up to you on the sidewalk or meet you in the parking lot and walk with you to the front door. In the case of a blockade or other particularly aggressive harassment, you may see a large group of volunteers, 10, 20, or more. If antichoice picketers are trying to give you literature or stop you from entering the clinic, several escorts may get between you and the protesters, or they may form a circle around you and keep you surrounded until you are safely inside the building. If picketers are trying to photograph or videotape women entering the building, an escort may put a shirt or jacket over your head and guide you to the door.

Clinics that are picketed regularly often have client escorts, and in some cases, you may be told ahead of time to look for them outside the building. In situations of heavy harassment, it may be difficult to tell who is a prochoice volunteer and who is not, so be sure to find out how to rec-ognize the escorts. Ask what they will be wearing and what they will say when they come up to you.

CLINIC ACCESS AND "BUBBLE" LAWS

Clinic access and "bubble" laws are intended to protect the safety of clinic patients and staff, as well as protesters' free speech rights under the First Amendment.

The Freedom of Access to Clinic Entrances Act (FACE) passed in 1994 makes it illegal for anyone to use force, the threat of force, or a physical obstruction to intentionally injure, intimidate, or interfere with clinic pa-tients or staff. It provides heavy criminal penalties—fines and prison sen-tences—for vandalism, physical assault, and shootings. Individuals and clinics can also sue protesters for civil damages. While FACE has been credited with decreasing clinic violence in general, it can only be enforced by federal agents, such as U.S. marshals and attorneys. Local police responding to a clinic blockade cannot use it to arrest protesters.

In such instances, state and local laws are needed. Twelve states have passed clinic access laws similar to FACE but more narrowly written. They outlaw blockades and certain kinds of physical and verbal harassment. Punishment for violators is less severe; an initial violation may be a misdemeanor with a fine of up to $1,000 and 60 to 90 days in jail.

Individual cities have also passed so-called bubble laws in response to particular picketing situations at local clinics. These laws usually establish a safety zone, or "bubble," around individuals entering a clinic, or the clinic itself. Picketers must stay outside this zone, usually 8 to 15 feet for individuals and 15, 30, or 100 feet or more for clinics. Local ordinances have also been used to set noise levels for antichoice protests or ban groups from picketing the homes of individual doctors or clinic staff. Antichoice groups have contested bubble laws in court, and certain provisions of the laws have been ruled unconstitutional. Bans against picketing doctors' homes have been overturned, and safety zones around clinics and individuals have been reduced.

Note: Where bubble laws establish personal safety zones around individual women, the zone may only be "activated"—considered legally valid— if you tell picketers to stay away from you or wear a sign that lets them know you don't want to speak with them. For example, you could wear or carry a sign that says, "Prochoice. Don't speak to me." If you don't say anything or wear a sign, picketers have the right to approach you, talk to you, and try to give you antichoice literature.

Again, the impact of clinic access and bubble laws often depends on how well they are being enforced, which varies widely from state to state and clinic to clinic. Your provider will be able to tell you if your state or city has a clinic access or bubble law and whether the laws are being enforced.

GETTING IN SAFELY: WHAT YOU CAN DO

☑ Even if you are faced with intense harassment, a few simple, effective strategies can help you get inside a clinic quickly and safely. Here are recommendations from providers and client escorts.

Be Prepared

When you make your appointment, ask if the clinic is likely to be picketed and what to expect. How many protesters usually show up? What do they do? Will client escorts be outside? If you've never been to the clinic before, ask if the building has a private parking lot, garage, or back entrance you can use to get in without crossing a picket line or walking by sidewalk counselors.

Get a Weekday Appointment

At most clinics, picketing is heaviest on weekends. More picketers show up, and they tend to be more aggressive. If possible, make your appointment for a weekday. Harassment is more likely to be minimal—a few picketers or none at all.

Don't Drive Your Own Car

If you are concerned about picketers writing down your license plate number, don't drive your own car. Borrow a friend's or ask someone to give you a ride—don't worry, it is unlikely the antis will bother your friend. If driving your own car is the only choice, leave it in a public lot or shopping center a short distance from the clinic and take a cab to and from the building.

Get Dropped off at the Front Door

If you park your car on the street and walk to the clinic's front door, picketers will have more time and opportunity to harass you, even if you're with a partner or other support person. Instead, ask your provider for the drop-off point nearest the front door, and have your partner or friend let you out there. In many cases, the front door or nearest client escort may be only a few steps away. Your partner or support person can then park the car and come in after you.

Don't Stop Your Car for Picketers

If picketers are trying to block the clinic's parking lot, keep your windows rolled up, don't talk to them, and *don't stop*, even if they stand directly in front of your car. Stop only if protesters are lying down in the driveway or parking lot entrance; in all other instances, drive slowly, but keep moving forward. Providers and client escorts say picketers will move when they see that you are not going to stop.

Drown Them Out!

If you don't want to hear what picketers are saying, drown them out! When driving into the clinic's parking lot, play your car radio—loud. If you have to cross a picket line, bring a Walkman or boom box and pump up the volume so that you don't have to hear their slogans or other verbal harassment.

Don't Be Polite! Ignore Them!

Many women have been raised to be polite and considerate, and in some cases, they may think they should stop and listen to sidewalk counselors or take antichoice literature, whether they want to or not. Others may be friendly when picketers approach, not realizing that stopping for even a moment means exposing themselves to verbal or physical harassment.

Remember, these people are *not* being polite; they are deliberately invading your privacy and violating your rights. They may even be breaking the law. *Ignore them!* You do not have to take their literature or listen to them at all. If picketers approach you as you are walking toward the building, let them know clearly and unmistakably that you want to be left alone. If a group of picketers tries to surround you or block your way, keep your head and arms down and push your way through or around them.

Note: Whatever protesters do or say, no matter how aggressive or violent they become, do *not* push, shove, hit, or threaten them in any way. If you, your partner, or any friend or family member pushes or hits a protester—even in self-defense—other picketers may claim you have "assaulted" that person. If police are present, they may demand that you be arrested. If picketers push, grab, or physically threaten you or anyone entering the clinic with you, report the incident immediately to a client escort or other clinic staff.

Pretend You're a Client Escort

Another way to ward off aggressive picketers is to pretend you're a client escort instead of a client. "The antis are at the clinic to harass clients," says Laura Weide, a long-time prochoice activist and client escort in California. "They don't really harass the people who are there to escort, or at least, they don't try to stop them from getting into the clinic. If you see a bunch of antis coming toward you and they ask if you're a client, say no. Act like you're a prochoice person; tell them you're here to keep the clinic open, put your fist in the air, and start walking toward the clinic." Weide adds that during blockades or other intense harassment, client escorts may "disguise" a woman and help her get into the clinic by having her wear an escort T-shirt, vest, or armband.

Don't Argue with Them

Going through an antichoice picket line in silence may leave some women feeling powerless, angry, or victimized. Yell back or let the protesters know how you feel if you want, but *don't* try to argue or debate with them. Explaining the prochoice point of view or telling them about your situation will not change their minds, and in many cases, it may only make a tense or uncomfortable situation worse.

Keep in mind that when you yell at picketers, they usually yell back, only louder (see **Yelling Back: Kim's Story**, p. 112). Again, the best way to demoralize picketers is to show them you don't care what they are doing by laughing or ignoring them.

Annie was in her thirties and the divorced mother of a school-age daughter when she became pregnant and decided to have an abortion. An active member of local prochoice groups, she was not surprised or threatened when protesters tried to stop her and her boyfriend from entering the clinic. "I had to go inside for my appointment, so we just walked through the line" said Annie. "My boyfriend is also completely prochoice, so I left him outside and said, 'Sic 'em, hon.' He walked up to the protesters and said, 'You know, seeing all you people out here really inspires me. It makes me want to write a big check to the clinic.' Then he laughed and came inside."

If You Can't Get into the Building, Call the Clinic

When you make your appointment, the clinic should give you a telephone number to call in case you are going to be late or can't get into the building. Be sure you have this number with you when you leave for your appointment. If the building is being blockaded, or you don't feel safe trying to get inside, go to a nearby pay phone and call the clinic. Your appointment will be rescheduled, or a security guard or client escort will be sent out to help you get inside the building. If a guard or escort is sent, ask the clinic for the person's name, what she or he looks like, and an identifying piece of clothing. If the person meeting you will be driving a car, find out its make, color, and license plate number.

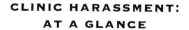

CLINIC HARASSMENT:
AT A GLANCE

• Antichoice protesters have a right to free speech; they don't have a right to harass you. Federal, state, and local laws now make it illegal to blockade a clinic or try to injure or intimidate anyone entering a clinic.

• Prayer vigils, picketing, and sidewalk counseling are the most common types of clinic harassment. Picketers may also try to write down your license plate number and find out your name and address.

• Find out ahead of time if the clinic is expecting picketers. Ask how many to expect and what they usually do.

• Also find out about the clinic's security procedures, where to park, and whether to look for guards or client escorts. Escorts often wear clothes that make them easy to spot, such as brightly colored vests, hats, or T-shirts.

• Try to schedule your appointment for a weekday or other time when picketing or other forms of harassment are less likely to occur.

• If you are concerned about your license plate number being written down by picketers, don't drive your car to the clinic. Get a friend to drive you, borrow a car, or park your car a short distance from the clinic and take a cab.

• If the clinic is being picketed when you arrive, do whatever you can to get into the building quickly and safely. *Don't be polite!* Do not stop your car for picketers. Don't talk or debate with them. Do not accept literature.

• No matter how aggressive or threatening picketers get, *don't* push or shove them back or threaten them in any way, even in self-defense. You could get arrested.

+ If you are harassed by picketers and feel upset or angry, ask to speak with a counselor. Don't get mad at clinic staff.

+ Make sure you have a contact number for the clinic. If the entrance is blocked or you do not feel safe trying to get into the building, go to a pay phone and call the clinic immediately.

8

TAKING CARE OF YOURSELF

Read this chapter for information on how to take care of yourself emotionally and physically during an unplanned pregnancy.

An unplanned pregnancy can be one of the most terrifying, confusing, and truly harrowing experiences any woman can have. From the first instance of morning sickness or breast tenderness, your body feels invaded and out of control. You can't eat or sleep, you're nauseated or throwing up every morning, if not all day, and your hormones are seriously out of whack. You're angry with your boyfriend, and yourself, for getting pregnant in the first place. To top it all off, you may desperately want to talk with someone but may not be sure who to trust. Will your husband support your decision? Will your folks yell at you? Will your best friend suddenly turn into an antichoice zealot and blab it all over school or the office? Are you even sure what you want to do?

Having an abortion can be stressful for many reasons, the least of which is the stigma that continues to surround and silence women who choose to terminate unplanned pregnancies. Women who have abortions are still considered to have done something "bad" or "wrong." They are not supposed to talk about their needs or experiences, at least not publicly, and they are not supposed to feel good about themselves before or after the procedure.

The consequences of such attitudes can be painful and frustrating. Faced with an unplanned pregnancy, some women may neglect and isolate themselves at a time when good care and support are most essential. Abortion is a medical procedure, and your physical and emotional health can affect the outcome. If you are in good physical condition before an abortion, complications are less likely, and your recovery will be quicker.

Similarly, providers say that women who take good care of themselves emotionally—who talk about their feelings and ask for support from friends and family—are more likely to be comfortable with their decisions and see the abortion as a positive experience.

This chapter contains basic information on how to reduce the emotional and physical stress of an unplanned pregnancy. It covers:

⬧ The emotional experience of an unplanned pregnancy and abortion: what you may or may not be feeling

⬧ Why support is so important, and figuring out who to talk to

⬧ The dangers of self-induced abortion

⬧ The physical symptoms of early pregnancy, and what you can do about them

---

THE "ANGUISH" OF ABORTION: FACT AND FICTION

In recent years, media images of women who have abortions have focused almost exclusively on the "anguish" of the decision to terminate an unplanned or unwelcome pregnancy. Antichoice groups have also presented a distorted picture of women's emotional needs, claiming that women who have abortions will suffer from "postabortion trauma syndrome" and remain psychologically "damaged" by guilt, shame, and remorse for years following the procedure.

While the majority of women do think carefully about whether or not to have an abortion, most will make their decision in a relatively short time—usually within a few days or weeks of having a pregnancy test. Temporary feelings of anxiety or sadness can be expected at this time, but in general most women feel comfortable with their decisions. They are relieved after having an abortion and return to their normal lives within a few days or weeks.

"A woman is usually the best gauge of how she'll do emotionally," says Anne Baker, head of counseling at a clinic in Illinois. "If you think, 'I'm going to be able to cope with this,' you will. Just knowing that, or having that attitude, can make a big difference in how you feel."

YOUR EMOTIONS: WHAT TO EXPECT

For most women, an unplanned pregnancy is a crisis that may trigger a range of conflicting and contradictory emotions. Some women know instantly what they want to do, while others may feel excited, guilty, or confused all at the same time. The decision to continue or terminate a pregnancy may be especially difficult if it becomes tangled with other issues in a woman's life, for example, education and career plans or how to deal with an abusive partner or parent.

Focusing on your own emotions may seem difficult at this time, but it is essential. *Find someone you can trust—a partner, friend, or clinic counselor—and talk to them.* Both providers and women who have had abortions agree that getting emotional support is the most important and helpful thing any woman can do to minimize the stress and isolation of an unplanned pregnancy and think clearly about what she really wants to do (see **Who to Tell**, p. 130).

Remember also that every woman's experience at this time will be different. There is no right or wrong way to think or feel. How any woman approaches the situation will depend on a range of factors, such as her cultural or ethnic background, career and family status, plans for the future, and spiritual or religious beliefs.

Powerlessness

However many times you may have thought about what you would do if you became pregnant and wanted an abortion, the actual experience may leave you feeling powerless and out of control of your life. For some women, feelings of powerlessness become so overwhelming that waiting a week or two for an appointment seems intolerable (see **Chapter 10**). Physical symptoms, like morning sickness and breast tenderness, can make you feel even more out of control, especially if you've never been pregnant before (see **Your Body: What to Expect**, p. 134). A woman may also feel desperate if she wants an abortion but thinks she won't be able to get one because she can't get to a clinic, doesn't have the money, or lives in a state with an informed consent or parental notification or consent law (see **Self-Induced Abortion: Don't Do It!**, p. 133).

Isolation

Women who have abortions frequently speak about feeling isolated and unable to talk with anyone about their experiences and emotions. Women whose partners or parents are not supportive often feel especially alone, as do women living in small towns or rural areas, where confidentiality is difficult to maintain and any trip to a clinic can cause raised eyebrows and uncomfortable questions. Deciding who to tell may be an additional source of stress and isolation. A negative response from someone you have always trusted—a friend, local clergy, or family doctor—can be particularly hurtful and leave you feeling even more cut off from your usual support system (see **Who to Tell**, p. 130).

Guilt

However certain and determined a woman may be about her decision to have an abortion, she may still have to grapple with feelings of guilt, shame, and selfishness. Teenagers may feel guilty about being sexually active and having to tell their parents they are pregnant. Women who have had unprotected sex may feel ashamed, and a bit foolish, about being careless and getting "caught." For those who have been raised to believe that abortion is bad or immoral, even thinking about terminating a pregnancy may feel like an unforgivable "sin." Women who already have children and know both the joys and burdens of parenting may feel selfish and "unnatural." You may even feel guilty because you don't feel ashamed or bad and think you should.

Anger

During an unplanned pregnancy, a woman may find herself in many situations that make her feel angry or frustrated. When she first finds out she is pregnant, she may feel angry because she and her partner didn't use birth control or the methods they used didn't work. Later, she may be angry if a friend or family member does not support her decision to have an abortion or pressures her to terminate the pregnancy when she doesn't want to. Lack of communication between partners or family members can also be a source of anger: for example, if you wake up feeling nauseated every morning, and your partner is insensitive to your need for extra help and emotional support.

Surprise and Excitement

Not all emotions connected to an unplanned pregnancy will be negative. If you have never been pregnant before, or even if you have, you may be surprised and excited when you first find out you are pregnant. Women in their teens and early twenties often think they will never get pregnant, and a positive pregnancy test may represent a sudden and unexpected affirmation of their ability to have children. Their first thought may be "Hey, I can really do this!" If a woman has tried to get pregnant but has been unable to, she may also be initially excited and then confused if she feels continuing the pregnancy is not possible because of personal circumstances, such a recent divorce or the financial stress of a sick relative.

Sadness

For some women, the fetus represents a potential life or unique spirit, and the decision to have an abortion, however certain, may trigger feelings of sadness, loss, and grief. If a woman has always wanted a child but is unable to continue a pregnancy, she may feel that she will never have another chance. Women having second-trimester abortions may have started to form an emotional bond with the fetus and may feel physically empty after the procedure. Feelings of grief and loss may also be common for women who already have children or would like to have a child with their current partner but feel that the timing of the pregnancy is not right.

Ambivalence

Some women may feel ambivalent about deciding to have an abortion, even when they have considered all their options and know that terminating the pregnancy is the best choice for them. Women who are actively prochoice may find the experience of unplanned pregnancy more complex and upsetting than they expected. Similarly, an unwelcome pregnancy may force women who have always opposed abortion to re-examine their values. For women in their thirties or early forties who have never had children, an unplanned pregnancy may seem like their last chance, and they may be especially conflicted if they still feel that abortion is their only or best choice.

Numbness

Some women close down emotionally or "numb out" during an unplanned pregnancy. They are afraid of their emotions or simply don't want to deal with them. Providers say that women who numb out focus almost exclusively on the practical details of having an abortion—getting a pregnancy test, finding a clinic, and making whatever other arrangements may be necessary. They usually say they just want to "get the whole thing over with" and rarely want to speak with a counselor before or after the procedure.

Note: Just because you don't want to speak with a counselor doesn't mean you have numbed out or are not dealing with your emotions. Many women do talk about their feelings with friends and family, and by the time they get to a clinic, they are completely comfortable with their decisions. Providers also recognize that for some women, numbing out "works"—it gets them through a difficult situation—especially if they feel unable to ask anyone they know for help or are facing other crises in their lives. In such instances, feelings about the pregnancy and abortion may surface at a later date—months or even years afterward. This is normal and natural. It is *not* "postabortion trauma syndrome," as antichoice groups have claimed. However, repressed emotions can be powerful and upsetting, and you may wish to speak with a partner, friend, or counselor at this time.

FEELING GOOD ABOUT YOURSELF AND YOUR DECISION

For most women the decision to have an abortion is a survival decision. The pregnancy is unplanned or unwelcome, and carrying it to term would risk their own or their family's well-being: physical, emotional, or economic. Again, this may be a difficult or sad decision, but many women find that having an abortion can also be a positive experience, an opportunity for personal change and growth.

Lucy was a freshman in college and away from home and her church-going parents for the first time when she became pregnant and decided to have an abortion. It was, she recalls, a turning point in her life. "Until then, it was always my parents telling me what to do," she said. "Even the college I chose, I went to because my dad wanted me to. Having the abortion was the first time I made a decision just for me. I was taking control of my life. I was determining where my future was going to be. Today, I look back at that, and I'm really proud of myself. I was doing it for me, and it made me feel really good."

To ensure that you feel comfortable about your decision, providers say to take all the time—and if possible, get all the support—you need, even if it means waiting a week or two or having a second-trimester procedure.

Keep in mind also that many women have not been raised to think of themselves as decision makers and rarely give themselves credit or reward themselves for making hard decisions. Whether you choose to terminate or continue your pregnancy, *you have made the decision that is right for you, and you deserve to feel good about it.*

Here are some of the things you can do to ensure that you feel good or at least comfortable about the decision you make.

Clarify

Women's feelings about unplanned pregnancy and abortion are often rooted in social stereotypes and attitudes that may have little to do with their current beliefs and situations. Simply put, just because you feel guilty or selfish does not mean that you are. Talking about your emotions may help you think clearly about your present circumstances and put them in a more positive and realistic perspective.

For example, if a woman is feeling guilty because she thinks she is putting herself or her interests first, she may need to differentiate between selfishness and healthy self-interest. Having an abortion is not selfish if it means you will be able to get a good education or take care of the family and children you already have. Similarly, if you are initially excited about being pregnant, you may need to differentiate between the positive feelings you have about your ability to get pregnant and whether you want to continue or terminate this particular pregnancy.

Vent!

Women who feel overwhelmed or confused by their emotions may not only feel badly about themselves, they may repress, misdirect, or act out their feelings in unhealthy or self-destructive ways. They may start yelling or crying over small, seemingly inconsequential matters, or they may turn to drugs, alcohol, or other compulsive behaviors to help them numb out or relax. While often understandable, this kind of behavior not only increases the stress of an unplanned pregnancy; it may also obscure or further confuse your emotions and options.

Venting or expressing your emotions will help you feel more in control and allow you to focus on what's really bothering you. Safe, healthy ways to vent include writing in a journal; talking with a supportive, nonjudgmental friend; having a good cry, laugh, or temper tantrum; taking a walk; or getting more vigorous physical exercise if you feel up to it.

Note: If a woman has used alcohol or drugs—prescription or "recreational"—before or right after finding out she is pregnant, she may feel she has to have an abortion because of potential genetic damage to the fetus. While long-term alcohol or drug use can harm fetal development, having a few drinks, or even occasionally taking drugs, in the first few weeks of pregnancy may not cause any damage to the fetus. If you are concerned about your alcohol or drug consumption and the effect it may have on the fetus, you should speak with a doctor or genetic counselor. Referrals and frank, unbiased information on fetal development are available from most providers.

Focus on What You Need Right Now

As noted, feelings about an unplanned pregnancy can become tangled and confused with other issues in a woman's life, such as a failed or abusive relationship or present or future career plans. If this is your situation, try to focus on what you need right now to make a decision that feels comfortable for you.

"You need to get all the garbage out of the way and stick with basic questions," says Eileen Tamsky, a counselor at a clinic in Missouri. "What needs to happen for you? Who do you need to speak to? What do you need to do? What information do you need? If you're worried about being able to get pregnant again, do you need to talk to a doctor for a second opinion? Are you making assumptions about what your partner does or doesn't want? Do you need to go to this person and say, 'Look, how do you really feel about this?' Focus on what you feel, not necessarily what you think."

Pamper Yourself

Providers also encourage women to pamper themselves during an unplanned pregnancy. Take time to relax—even if it's only for a few minutes a day—and do something that makes you feel good. Take a walk, take a bubble bath, get a new haircut, go out to dinner with friends, or just curl up with a good book.

WHO TO TELL

While having someone to talk with can ease the stress and isolation of an unplanned pregnancy, a woman's need for support must often be balanced with her desire for confidentiality. You may want to share your decision to terminate or continue the pregnancy with a few people, but still not want others to know. You may also be uncertain about who it is safe to tell. In such instances, trust your instincts, and remember that a good support person will both respect your privacy and listen to you without criticizing or trying to tell you what to do.

If you are unsure if the people close to you will be supportive, check out their feelings about abortion before you tell them. Mention that you recently saw a magazine article or television show on abortion—make up something if you haven't—and watch how they react. If they express strong antichoice opinions, such as "I don't believe in abortion" or "Women who have abortions are careless or selfish," you may wish to confide in someone else.

Similarly, if you are considering talking about your decision with your minister, rabbi, or family doctor, try to find out if this person is prochoice. Call your church, synagogue, or doctor's office anonymously, and ask if they can refer you to a clinic that performs abortions. In the case of a doctor, you can also ask if she or he is a provider. Again, if the answer to any of these questions is no, you may wish to speak with someone else.

Keep in mind that the decision to confide in other people always involves some risks—and surprises. Laura was at college in a small New England town when she became pregnant and decided to have an abortion. Home for a holiday break before the procedure, she confided in two friends and recalls being surprised by both their reactions. "An old boyfriend was really wonderful," said Laura. "It was very surprising because of all my friends, he was the one I figured would go absolutely nuts and tell me I had to have the baby. He asked me when my appointment was and if I needed any help, and he sent me flowers two days later. We've become even better friends since then. Another friend, my best friend since second grade, went the opposite way. I figured she'd be very supportive, but she got righteous and judgmental, and we haven't spoken much since then."

Women under 18 may need to be especially careful about who they tell or ask for help. Teachers or school counselors may think that they are required to tell your principal or parents that you are pregnant, even though in most cases a teen's confidentiality is protected by law. Think twice also before telling a classmate—especially if it's someone you've known for only a few weeks or months—even if she or he "swears" to keep your secret (see **Chapter 3**).

If You Want to Speak to a Counselor

According to providers, about 5 to 10 percent of the women they see may be ambivalent about continuing or terminating an unplanned pregnancy and may need additional help or counseling either before or after an abortion. For example, exploring all your options may not seem possible when your partner is threatening to leave you if you do or don't have an abortion. In other instances, the problem may not be the decision itself but feelings of isolation or lack of support from friends or family.

If you are uncertain about your decision or just need someone to talk with, pre- and postabortion counseling is available at most clinics and is usually free and confidential. Counseling sessions last about an hour, and during this time, you will be encouraged to talk about your emotions and what you need to make a decision that feels right for you. Counselors may also give you pamphlets or worksheets with questions and writing exercises that will help you consider all your options. If you are unable to come to the clinic—either because you live too far away or can't arrange transportation—counseling by phone can usually be arranged. Some clinics also offer family counseling sessions for women and their partners or teens and their parents.

Note: At most clinics, pre- and postabortion counseling is limited to one or two sessions. If a woman needs more counseling—for example, for relationship or drug or alcohol problems—most clinics will provide referrals to an appropriate therapist or community organization.

Religious or Spiritual Counseling

For some women, an unplanned pregnancy can raise questions or conflicts related to their religious or spiritual beliefs. If you belong to a church or religious group that is publicly antichoice, you may feel cut off and alienated from the friends and clergy you have always relied on for support. In other instances, doubt and ambivalence about an abortion decision may be rooted in childhood beliefs about God and religion, even if you haven't been to church for many years.

If you are seeking spiritual counseling but feel unable to talk with local clergy or simply do not belong to a church or synagogue, call the **Religious Coalition for Reproductive Choice** (RCRC). The coalition has chapters in many states and refers women to prochoice clergy who have received special training in pre- and postabortion counseling. One-hour counseling sessions are free and confidential; and where possible, you will be matched with prochoice clergy from your specific religious group or denomination. Your clinic should be able to refer you to the RCRC office closest to you; or you can call the National Abortion Federation referral line at 800-772-9100. Individual clinics may also be able to refer you to prochoice clergy in your area.

SELF-INDUCED ABORTION: DON'T DO IT!

✔ The desperation, anxiety, and powerlessness women feel during an unplanned pregnancy can, and too often still do, lead many to attempt to induce their own abortions. Prior to legalization in the United States, an estimated 1,000 to 5,000 women per year were dying from illegal abortions. Internationally, 200,000 women per year continue to die from botched illegal abortions.

While legalization has made abortion safe and more accessible in the United States, in recent years stories of self-induced abortion have again begun to surface. Coat hangers, chopsticks, knitting needles, and household chemicals like Drano and lye are again being used by women who think they can't afford an abortion and by teenagers who are afraid to tell their parents. In isolated cases, women desperate to induce their own abortions have even thrown themselves off moving vehicles.

Self-induced abortions do *not* work, and the complications they cause are serious and lethal. Possible complications include uncontrolled bleeding, toxic infections, lacerations of the cervix and uterus, uterine perforations, and death. Damage to the cervix and uterus can result in sterility, and swallowing household chemicals can burn out your stomach lining and cause permanent damage to your digestive system.

If you are thinking about trying to induce your own abortion, call a prochoice clinic in your area or the NAF or Planned Parenthood referral lines (see **Chapter 1**). However hopeless your situation may seem, these organizations can help you get a medically safe abortion. *If you or someone you know has tried to induce an abortion and is having severe cramps, bleeding, a high fever, vomiting, diarrhea, or other signs of possible complications, go immediately to a hospital emergency room.*

Herbal Abortion

Since the 1970s, several books have been published that describe the use of herbs and plants for inducing abortions. A recent example, *Herbal*

Abortion by Uni M. Tiamat, provides detailed instructions on how to prepare herbal teas and tinctures that, the author states, she has used herself to terminate pregnancies safely and effectively early in the first trimester.

Historical and anecdotal evidence suggests that certain herbs and plants can, in fact, induce abortions. *However, the procedures and methods used are neither safe nor reliable.* **Some herbs are highly toxic and, when taken improperly, can cause heavy cramping and bleeding, nausea, diarrhea, high blood pressure, heart failure, and death.**

Linda, a teenager who tried herbs before getting a surgical abortion, says 2 weeks of taking herbal teas left her sick, scared, and still pregnant. "I read some books about herbal abortion and decided to try it," she recalls. "I would go home from school everyday and make herbal teas. I had cramps and threw up, but nothing else happened."

Herbs are also associated with birth defects and other damage to the fetus, and if an herbal abortion is not successful, the pregnancy should still be terminated. "I've counseled several women who did herbs and then wanted to continue their pregnancies, and I had to talk them out of it," says Stacey Haugland, the director of a clinic in Montana. "There's too much risk to the fetus. If you try herbs and they don't work, you need to go to a clinic and have a surgical abortion."

YOUR BODY: WHAT TO EXPECT

The physical symptoms of pregnancy are one of the least discussed, but most stressful, aspects of an unplanned pregnancy. No matter how quickly you make your decision, the fact remains that for a few weeks or months you will be pregnant, and your body will go through some of the physical changes associated with early pregnancy. Morning sickness, breast tenderness, and fatigue are women's most common complaints, and emotional isolation at this time can make any physical discomfort even worse.

Taking care of yourself before an abortion is essential, and whether your pregnancy is planned or unplanned, symptoms should be treated the same. There are simple, effective ways to ease physical discomfort. Information and advice on how to minimize symptoms is also available from most clinics. Keep in mind that every pregnancy is different, and specific symptoms and how they respond to treatment may vary from woman to woman and pregnancy to pregnancy.

Morning Sickness

Morning sickness is often the first and most unpleasant sign that a woman is pregnant. Symptoms range from general lightheadedness or queasiness to severe nausea and vomiting. Standing, eating, and other normal physical activities may be difficult, if not impossible. Some women do seem to be more affected in the morning, but bouts of dizziness and nausea may occur at any time of the day.

Ellen, who had an abortion in her mid-twenties, remembers a particularly difficult 2 weeks when even standing up made her feel sick. "I had just been promoted to a new job at work when I got pregnant," said Ellen. "So the timing was not particularly good. I never threw up, but if I was on my feet for more than five or ten minutes, I'd get queasy and lightheaded and would have to sit or lie down. I called it 'day sickness' because it literally went on all day. It got so bad that I couldn't function at the office. The last two days before the abortion, I called in sick and stayed home."

While the exact cause of morning sickness is still unknown, changes in reproductive and digestive hormones appear to be the likely culprits. Symptoms usually begin between the second and eighth week of pregnancy and vary widely, and wildly, from woman to woman. Attacks of dizziness or nausea can be triggered by certain foods and smells or simply by getting out of bed or standing up too quickly. Most women will experience only intermittent or moderate nausea, but for a very small number, the vomiting and inability to eat may become so severe that hospitalization can be required.

While morning sickness may not be avoidable—it affects about 85 percent of all pregnant women—some of its more disruptive and uncomfortable aspects can be minimized. Here are some of the things you can do:

Graze   The best way to reduce nausea and vomiting is to try to keep a little food in your stomach at all times. Most providers suggest grazing—eating several small, light meals over the course of the day, instead of three big ones. Foods high in protein and complex carbohydrates—fresh fruits and vegetables, wholewheat crackers and breads—are recommended, but in general, eat whatever you can keep down.

Eat before You Get out of Bed in the Morning   Keep crackers or a piece of bread or dry toast by your bed and eat them before you get up. Another remedy for early morning queasiness is sipping ginger ale, coke syrup over ice, or ginger or chamomile tea while you're still in bed. When you do get up, move slowly. Sudden or abrupt movement may bring on nausea or vomiting, especially if your stomach is empty.

Drink Plenty of Fluids   Women experiencing moderate to severe vomiting may be at risk for dehydration. If you are vomiting a lot, be sure to drink plenty of fluids—water, juice, or soups—whatever you can keep down. Try to sip throughout the day—don't guzzle or chug—and limit what you drink during meals. Putting too much in your stomach too fast could trigger more nausea. If you are having trouble with fluids, try eating fresh fruits and vegetables with a high water content, such as lettuce, melon, and citrus fruit.

Avoid Strong Smells   During pregnancy, your sense of smell may become more acute and sensitive, and odors that don't normally bother you may trigger sudden attacks of queasiness or nausea. Spicy foods, tobacco smoke, or other strong smells may be particularly hard to tolerate. Avoid whatever you can. If the smell of certain foods makes you nauseous, don't eat or cook them, even if it means your boyfriend or family goes without a favorite dish for a week or two.

Take Vitamin B$_6$ Small doses of vitamin B$_6$ can help reduce nausea and vomiting for some women. The recommended dosage is 25 to 50 milligrams a day and should be taken in addition to other vitamins.

Ask Your Pharmacist about Antinausea Medications   Antinausea medications, such as Nauzene, Bonine, and Dramamine, are available over the counter at most drugstores. Sea-Bands, 1-inch bands worn on both wrists, are also effective against nausea and are available at drugstores and marine shops.

Note: *Check with your provider before taking any antinausea vitamins or drugs.* You should take them only if you are absolutely certain you are going to have an abortion. High doses of vitamin B$_6$ can cause neurological damage to a developing fetus, and most antinausea medications are not recommended for pregnant women. If you ask a pharmacist for an antinausea drug, be sure to tell her or him that you are pregnant, and read any instructions or warnings on the label carefully.

Breast Tenderness

Hormonal changes in early pregnancy may cause your breasts to swell and become extremely tender. Women who sleep on their side or stomach may suddenly find these positions uncomfortable, and certain forms of exercise, such as jogging and aerobics, may also increase sensitivity and soreness.

For tender or sore breasts, wear a good supportive bra, even if it means going out and buying a new one. Find a bra that fits well and keeps your breasts close to your body—like a sport or jogging bra—and wear it all the time, in bed as well as during the day. Taking vitamin E and cutting down on foods and liquids with caffeine, including chocolate, coffee, sodas, and black or other nonherbal teas, may also help decrease breast tenderness.

Fatigue

Being pregnant places heavy, unaccustomed demands on a woman's body. Some women find they tire easily or just feel listless. Pregnancy-related sleep disturbances can add to the problem. For example, frequent urination begins early in pregnancy for some women, and you may be getting up several times during the night for trips to the bathroom. Similarly, if you are nauseated in the mornings, you may be waking up earlier.

The treatment for pregnancy-related fatigue is simple, if not always convenient. Get extra rest. Accept that for a few weeks you may need to cut back on your normal levels of activity, and try to pace yourself. At home, ask your partner or a friend for help with housework, shopping, taking care of the kids, or other daily chores. If you have young children, take a nap with the kids instead of doing housework. Stay in a couple of nights a week and go to bed early. If repeated trips to the bathroom at night are keeping you up, try cutting back on fluids before you go to sleep.

At work, prioritize and delegate. Rest rather than run errands during your lunch hour, and if your company has an employee lounge, put your feet up and close your eyes for a few minutes. If part of your job is physically demanding or hard to do because of the pregnancy, see if you can work around it for a week or two or, again, ask for help.

Mood Swings

Mood swings are one of the more disruptive and frustrating symptoms of early pregnancy. Hormonal changes can and probably will affect your emotions, and there's not too much anyone can do about it.

Early pregnancy can feel like a particularly intense attack of premenstrual syndrome (PMS). You may find yourself feeling depressed, overly sensitive, or easily upset or angered. Mood swings may be abrupt and dramatic, and your mental concentration may also be affected.

Being aware of mood swings can help you feel more in control, and as with PMS, cutting caffeine and sugar may help level off the highs and lows. At the same time, don't discount your emotions—or let others discount them—just because they're hormonal. *The cause of your emotions has nothing to do with their validity*. If you need to cry, cry; if you're upset and want to yell, turn on some loud music and sing along at the top of your lungs (see **Feeling Good About Yourself and Your Decision**, p. 128).

Yeast Infections

Changes in vaginal pH levels—the acidity of the vagina—and an increase in vaginal discharge make some pregnant women highly susceptible to yeast infections. Unfortunately, most over-the-counter yeast medications are not recommended for use during pregnancy. If you are undecided about terminating or continuing the pregnancy, ask your provider about alternative treatments.

Eye Problems

Hormonal changes can also cause blurred vision, and women who wear hard contacts may suddenly find that their lenses are uncomfortable. Wear glasses instead. Your vision should return to normal after the abortion.

CONCEALING SYMPTOMS

For some women, treatment of pregnancy symptoms may be complicated by their need to conceal any signs of a missed period or ill health. Keeping crackers and tea by the bed may not be possible if you are a teenager living at home or have an abusive partner who doesn't know you're pregnant.

What any woman can and can't do will depend on her personal circumstances. To keep suspicions and uncomfortable questions to a minimum, your excuses should be vague and general. In a pinch, most women with morning sickness will say they have flu or stomach problems. A late period or small weight gain may be due to stress. If you have children, tell your boss you were late for work because of a sick kid.

SPOTTING AND CRAMPING

Spotting and cramping during early pregnancy are sometimes mistaken for a period, especially if a woman has an irregular menstrual cycle or is in denial about the pregnancy and is hoping it will go away if she ignores it. In fact, about one-third of all pregnant women experience minor bleeding and cramping. Spotting will be lighter than your normal menstrual period and should last only a day or two.

In a small number of cases, spotting may also be the first sign of a spontaneous abortion, or miscarriage, or of an ectopic pregnancy, when the fertilized egg becomes implanted in the fallopian tubes rather than the uterus. An ectopic pregnancy can be especially dangerous if undiagnosed: the pregnancy can burst the tube, and emergency surgery could be required.

If you are spotting, wear a pad instead of a tampon and monitor your bleeding carefully. Call your doctor or clinic if bleeding is heavy or continues for more than 3 days or if other symptoms such as dizziness, nausea, and heavy cramping or abdominal pain occur at the same time.

Another possibility is telling concerned or curious friends that you have recently started taking or switched birth control pills. The side effects of some pills are, ironically, similar to the symptoms of early pregnancy: nausea, breast tenderness, and weight gain.

WHEN WILL I START FEELING BETTER?

How fast pregnancy symptoms disappear depends on how long you've been pregnant. In many cases, women in the first trimester start to feel better within a few hours of the abortion. Their appetite returns, and nausea and other symptoms of morning sickness disappear. Breast tenderness, mood swings, and other sources of fatigue and discomfort may last until hormones drop back to prepregnancy levels, which can take a few days, a week, or longer.

Hormone levels are higher for women in the second trimester, and it may take longer for their bodies to return to normal. Women with swollen breasts may have to wait a week or two before they can sleep on their stomach or exercise comfortably. In a few cases, breast milk may develop. In such instances, continue to wear a supportive bra and don't touch or stimulate your nipples in any way. Your clinic can also give you medication to help dry up breast milk.

IF YOU DON'T HAVE SYMPTOMS

The early signs of pregnancy vary widely from woman to woman. Some women may have a few instances of minor discomfort; others may look and feel completely healthy.

If pregnancy symptoms are not a problem, providers recommend a normal schedule that includes nutritious food, regular exercise, and adequate rest. Even if your body doesn't appear to be changing physically, an unplanned pregnancy can be emotionally stressful and disruptive, and having a daily routine can help you feel more stable and in control of your life.

TAKING CARE OF YOURSELF: AT A GLANCE

+ While having an unplanned pregnancy can be a time of physical and emotional stress, it can also be an opportunity for personal change and growth. Right now, you need and deserve good care—from yourself and others.

+ An unplanned pregnancy can trigger a range of conflicting, contradictory, and very normal emotions, including powerlessness, guilt, anger, sadness, ambivalence, and even excitement.

+ *Coat hangers, Drano, and herbal teas can kill you!* No matter how depressed or desperate you feel, do not try to induce your own abortion.

+ *Don't go through it alone.* Find at least one person—a partner, friend, or family member—who can provide nonjudgmental support and will respect your privacy.

+ A woman's abortion decision can often become confused with other issues in her life—education, career plans, family, and relationships. Focus on what you are feeling and need right now.

+ Find healthy ways to express or vent your feelings: have a good cry, write in a journal, exercise, or talk with a friend.

+ Free pre- and postabortion counseling is available at most clinics, and referrals to counseling with prochoice clergy may also be available.

+ For morning sickness, try to keep something in your stomach at all times. Eat crackers or bread before you get out of bed and several small meals through the day. Vomiting can also cause dehydration, so be sure to drink plenty of fluids.

• For sore or tender breasts, make sure you have a good supportive bra and wear it at all times, even to bed.

• The best thing to do for pregnancy-related fatigue is sleep! If you're tired, ask for help, put your feet up, take naps, or stay in and go to bed early.

• If you have to hide morning sickness from friends and family, tell them you have flu or stomach problems. A missed period, extra weight gain, or mood swings can be due to stress.

• Most women are relieved after an abortion, but temporary feelings of sadness and grief are also normal. Talk with a supportive friend or counselor.

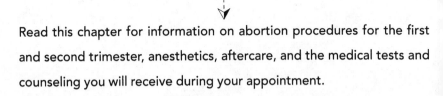

GETTING

AN ABORTION

Read this chapter for information on abortion procedures for the first and second trimester, anesthetics, aftercare, and the medical tests and counseling you will receive during your appointment.

Although abortion is one of the most common surgical procedures performed in the United States today, many people, women and men, continue to be confused or misinformed about what happens during an abortion and how safe the procedure really is. This lack of information often makes women nervous about going to a clinic or even calling for an appointment.

Having an abortion may feel especially intimidating if you have never been to a clinic or had a pelvic exam, as is often the case with teenagers or other women who do not have regular access to reproductive health care. Women may also be scared or upset if they have received inaccurate or distorted information about abortion from antichoice groups or phony clinics (see **Chapters 1 and 7**).

The truth is that a first-trimester abortion is twice as safe as a tonsillectomy, and prochoice clinics and doctors are recognized experts in the kind of outpatient surgery the procedure requires. Reputable providers—such as Planned Parenthood, feminist health centers, and members of the National Abortion Federation—maintain high professional standards so that every woman having an abortion can feel safe and well cared for. Information is an integral part of the comprehensive care these clinics offer. You can and should expect doctors, nurses, and other clinic staff to answer any questions you have about your pregnancy, your reproductive options, and the abortion procedure itself.

This chapter contains basic information on the abortion procedures now used by most providers and what to expect during your appointment. The topics covered include:

+ The safety of abortion

+ How to figure out how long you've been pregnant

+ The medical tests and counseling you will receive at the clinic

+ The anesthetics and pain medication commonly used for abortions

+ The vacuum aspiration method used for first-trimester abortions, and the dilation and evacuation method used in the second trimester

+ Postabortion care and counseling

ABORTION SAFETY: THE FACTS

Y Like any surgical procedure, abortion is not without its risks; however, antichoice claims of abortion causing infertility, breast cancer, or "postabortion trauma syndrome" are entirely unfounded. Since 1973, numerous studies have shown that abortion is safe and has little or no impact on women's health and fertility. Here are the facts.

+ *An estimated 1.3 million abortions are performed in the United States each year.* According to the U.S. Centers for Disease Control and Prevention, a vacuum aspiration abortion performed in the first 12 weeks of pregnancy is 7 times safer than giving birth and 100 times safer than an appendectomy. At present, about 54 percent of all abortions are performed before the 8th week of pregnancy, and 88 percent are done by the 12 week.

+ *The complication rate for abortion is extremely low.* For first-trimester procedures, the overall complication rate is less than 1 percent. Heavy bleeding, cramping, and infections occur in about 1 in 100 cases; perforation of the uterus occurs in 2 in 1,000. These complications are usually not serious and can be handled with a phone call or visit to your provider (see **Aftercare,** p. 155). For incomplete abortions, the procedure may have to be repeated—this is called a **resuction.** However, hospitalization is rare. The rate for hysterectomies (removal of the uterus) for all abortions is 1 in 1,000 cases, and death occurs in fewer than 1 in 200,000 cases.

+ *An abortion will not make you sterile or affect your ability to carry a future pregnancy to term.* According to the National Abortion and Re-

productive Rights Action League, medical studies from 21 countries
have found that women who have abortions routinely go on to have
normal, planned pregnancies and healthy babies. Abortion does not increase a woman's future risk for miscarriage or stillbirth, or for having
a low-birth-weight or congenitally deformed baby.

♦ *Abortion does not cause undue emotional trauma or postabortion
   trauma syndrome.* While an unplanned pregnancy can be stressful for
   many reasons, the American Psychological Association has stated that
   having an abortion does not cause women abnormal or long-term emotional trauma. The most common emotion women feel after an abortion is relief, and some find it can be a positive experience. Following
   the procedure, they feel stronger, more confident, and more in control
   of their lives.

♦ *Abortion does not increase a woman's risk for breast cancer.* According to the National Cancer Institute, there is no conclusive evidence of
   a link between abortion and breast cancer. About half of all current
   studies have found no connection, and where an increased risk has
   been indicated, it is equal to or less than other risk factors, such as living in a city or a woman's religion or marital status (see **Chapter 2**).

YOUR APPOINTMENT

▼ At most clinics, what happens before and after an abortion is just as
important as the procedure itself. The medical tests, information, and
counseling you receive are intended to make sure that your abortion is as
safe as possible and that you are fully informed about all your reproductive options and are comfortable with your decision. If you tell a counselor or any clinic staff that you are being pressured or feel ambivalent
about your decision, your abortion may be delayed and additional counseling recommended.

Specific procedures for preabortion tests and counseling will vary from
clinic to clinic. In general, here's what you can expect.

Calling the Clinic

When you call a clinic to make an appointment, you will be asked for basic personal information, including your name, address, phone number,
age, and the date of your last menstrual period. For many providers, the
first phone call is also a time to find out about you—your current situa-

HOW LONG HAVE I BEEN PREGNANT?

The kind of abortion you have will depend on how long you have been pregnant. During the first 12 to 14 weeks of pregnancy, the most commonly used procedure is vacuum aspiration, although a small number of clinics now offer early "medical" abortion using the abortion-inducing drugs mifepristone (RU-486) and methotrexate. For medical abortion, you must be no more than 7 or 8 weeks pregnant (see **Chapter 10**).

For abortions in the second trimester—after the 13th or 14th week and up to the 24th or 25th—the procedure is called dilation and evacuation, or D & E. Less than 1 percent of all abortions are performed after the 25th week; in most cases, late abortions are performed only if the fetus is deformed or if continuing the pregnancy would put a woman's life at risk. A very few doctors also perform intact dilations and extractions (IDEs) for abortions late in the second trimester, between 20 and 24 weeks (see **Chapter 11**).

To figure out how long you have been pregnant, do **not** count from the day you think you conceived. Most providers measure length of pregnancy from the first day of a woman's last normal menstrual period. If it is 2 months since the first day of your last period, you are 8 weeks pregnant; if it is 3 months, your doctor or clinic will probably say you are 12 or 13 weeks pregnant.

If you do not know the exact date of your last period, try to estimate and be sure to start with the first day of your last **normal** period. Some women have light spotting and cramping early in pregnancy and may miscalculate when their last period began (see **Chapter 8**). If you need to confirm the length of your pregnancy before your appointment—for example, if your provider only performs abortions up to 12 weeks, and you may be 13 weeks or more—an ultrasound scan should be arranged, either at the clinic or a local family planning center (see **Preabortion Medical Tests and Counseling,** p. 147).

tion, needs, and concerns—and answer any questions you have (see Chapter 1). Where necessary, information on state laws—informed consent, waiting periods, and parental involvement—will be discussed (see Chapters 2 and 3), and you will receive practical advice and instructions on how to prepare for your appointment. Depending on your situation, you could be on the phone for 5 to 10 minutes or over half an hour.

Write down any instructions or information you receive. Women are sometimes nervous or forgetful the day of their appointments, and if you leave an ID or insurance forms at home, your abortion may be delayed or even rescheduled. Here is some of the information you are likely to receive.

+ How long you can expect to be at the clinic.

+ Payment information. How much money you will need to bring, and what forms of payment the clinic accepts.

+ Whether you will need to bring a picture ID or any other forms of identification.

+ Whether you can eat, drink, or take prescription medications before your appointment.

+ The clinic's child care policy. Most providers strongly discourage women from bringing children with them, and in some cases it may be strictly forbidden (see **Chapter 6**).

+ Information on anesthetics and whether you will be able to drive home after the procedure or will need to have someone pick you up (see **Anesthetics**, p. 149).

+ What kind of clothes to wear. Loose, comfortable clothing is usually recommended; specifically, pants or a skirt you can slip on and off quickly and easily.

+ Whether the clinic is likely to be picketed by an antichoice group, and how to identify client escorts outside the clinic (see **Chapter 7**).

+ Other special instructions. Some providers request that women wear no jewelry or ask them to bring a few extrathick sanitary pads. Some also have special rules and surgical protocols for teens (see **If You Are under 18**, p. 147).

How Many Appointments Will I Need to Make?

The number of appointments you need to make will depend on the kind of procedure you are having, whether you live in a state with an informed consent law, and the policies and procedures of your clinic. In general, a vacuum aspiration procedure can be done in one appointment, although some clinics now require two: one for counseling and medical tests and a second, a day or two later, for the procedure itself. D & Es take two to four appointments, depending on how long you have been pregnant (see **Dilation and Evacuation**, p. 152). Informed consent laws may also mean an additional appointment for state-mandated counseling (see **Chapter 2**). Most appointments last 2 to 5 hours, and you can expect to spend at least some time in the waiting room.

Who to Bring

Most providers encourage women to have a support person with them at the clinic, and in some cases—for example, if you will not be able to drive after the procedure—it may be required. Friends or family members may be allowed to take part in your preabortion counseling session—after you have met with a counselor privately and then only if you say it's okay—however, they are usually not permitted in the procedure or recovery rooms. The person you ask to come with you should be someone who supports your decision fully and will be sensitive to your physical and emotional needs both before and after the abortion (see **Chapter 8**).

If you are having a second-trimester procedure or will be using a general anesthetic, you may need someone who can stay with you between appointments at the clinic and for up to 12 hours after the abortion (see **Anesthetics**, p. 149). When antichoice harassment is expected at the clinic, your support person should be someone who will not get angry or become violent if approached or yelled at by picketers (see **Chapter 7**).

Preabortion Medical Tests and Counseling

At most clinics, an abortion is preceded by a series of medical tests and counseling sessions. First, you will be asked to fill out a **medical history**

IF YOU ARE UNDER 18

Some providers have special rules or surgical protocols for minors, whether or not they are located in states with parental notification or consent laws. A signed parental consent form may be required at some clinics if you are under 16. In addition, a responsible adult over the age of 21 may have to come with you, especially if you live more than 2 hours from the clinic or are having a second-trimester abortion. If you are under 18, some providers may also require you to use a general anesthetic or laminaria, even if you are having a vacuum aspiration procedure. Again, this means you will need someone to come with you to the clinic, and if laminaria are being used, an extra appointment may be required (see **Anesthetics,** p. 149, and **Dilation and Evacuation**, p. 152).

form. The form contains important information your provider needs to perform your abortion safely and ensure you receive appropriate follow-up care: for example, if you are allergic to any drugs or are currently taking a prescription. Fill out the form as completely and accurately as possible.

After filling out the medical history, you will have **pregnancy and blood tests.** For the pregnancy test, a urine sample is used to determine or confirm the length of your pregnancy. Blood tests check for conditions, such as anemia or the Rh-negative blood factor, that could cause complications during or after your abortion. Blood samples may be collected by finger prick or by syringe.

Note: If a woman is Rh-negative, an abortion may result in the development of antibodies that can cause complications in future pregnancies. A shot of Rh immune globulin after the procedure ensures that antibodies do not develop and future pregnancies are not at risk. At some clinics, the shot is included in the price of the abortion; at others, it may be extra.

Preabortion counseling usually includes two components or sessions. First, you will meet privately with a specially trained counselor. No one else will be allowed in the room, and you will be encouraged to talk about your feelings and ask any questions you have. This session is intended to ensure a woman understands all her reproductive options, including adoption and carrying the pregnancy to term, and that no one is pressuring her to terminate or continue the pregnancy.

Next, you will be given information on the abortion procedure and its possible risks and complications (see **Abortion Safety,** p. 143, and **Abortion Procedures,** p. 150). This part of the counseling may be done individually or in a group with other women. At many clinics, partners and friends are also allowed to participate. Counselors often use posters or three-dimensional models to explain what happens during the procedure, and some may show you or let you handle surgical instruments such as speculums or dilating rods. Again, there will be time for questions, and at the end of the session you will be asked to sign a form that says you understand all the information you have received and want to have the abortion (see **Appendix 3**).

Ultrasound scans, or sonograms, are performed before an abortion to confirm how long a woman has been pregnant. In some cases, they may be done after the procedure to ensure the abortion is complete. Scans are similar to x-rays, except they use sound waves instead of radiation to create internal "pictures" of a person's body. Some clinics require sonograms only if a woman is close to or in her second trimester; others require them for all women.

Scans are usually performed by a nurse or other specially trained medical technician. If you are having a scan, you will be asked to remove your clothing from the waist down and lie on an examination table. You will be left alone to undress and given a paper sheet to cover your legs.

The ultrasound equipment includes a TV screen and a handheld scanning device that looks like a flashlight. When the scanner is moved over a woman's abdomen, it produces a grainy black-and-white image of her uterus and the fetus. In the early stages of pregnancy—less then 7 weeks—the scanner may be a smaller device, called a probe, that is inserted in your vagina. In most cases, the scan is completely painless.

You can decide whether or not you want to see the sonogram. At many clinics, ultrasound equipment is set up so that women are unable to see the screen. At others, screens are visible, and you will be told to turn your head or cover your eyes if you don't want to see the scan. Of course, if you want to see the sonogram, you will be allowed to, and a photo of the scan will be made for you if you request it. Again, the decision is yours, and you will not be judged or told what you should or shouldn't do.

Women's reactions to looking at sonograms vary widely. Some feel sad and upset, and a few may decide not to have an abortion. Others find that seeing the fetus actually confirms and strengthens their decision to terminate the pregnancy. In general, clinics are sensitive to women's reactions to scans and monitor individual women closely. If a woman feels upset or unsure about her decision after looking at a scan, additional counseling will be offered.

ANESTHETICS

At most clinics, a local anesthetic is included in the price of an abortion. The local numbs the cervix—the passage between the uterus and vagina—but does not put you to sleep or prevent cramping or other physical discomfort during the procedure. Many clinics also offer additional pain medication or sedatives, including tranquilizers, IV sedation or "twilight sleep," and general anesthetics. Information on the anesthetics available at your clinic will be discussed at the time you make your appointment and during your preabortion counseling session. At some clinics, additional medication costs extra—anywhere from $25 to $250.

Local anesthetics are usually recommended if you are having a vacuum aspiration abortion because they allow for quick recovery times—20 to 30 minutes—and are associated with low complication rates. Simply put, if you are awake during the abortion, you are more likely to be aware of any sharp or unusual pain, a sign of possible complications, and will be able to tell the doctor immediately. Tranquilizers have a similar effect: they help you feel more relaxed but do not reduce consciousness or physical discomfort during or after the procedure.

In most cases, women who use IV sedation or a general anesthetic will be semiconscious or unconscious during the abortion and will not remember it. Recovery time at the clinic ranges from 30 minutes to over an hour, and you may experience cramping and physical discomfort once the medication wears off. General anesthetics may also cause postabortion side effects, such as headaches, dizziness, and nausea.

If you use any extra medication—tranquilizers, IV sedation, or a general anesthetic—*you will not be allowed to drive after the procedure.* Some providers require women to bring a driver with them to the clinic; others simply want to make sure you have someone pick you up afterward. You may also need someone to stay with you for at least 12 hours after the procedure to ensure you have transportation back to the clinic in case any complications develop.

Note: *Combining any anesthetic with alcohol or street drugs may be dangerous.* Even if you are only planning to use a local anesthetic, you should *not* drink or take drugs before going to the clinic. If you do, tell your counselor or other clinic staff.

ABORTION PROCEDURES

Since the 1960s, the surgical methods used for abortions have been improved and refined by doctors and other providers, and special instruments and techniques have been developed to minimize women's discomfort and risk of complications. Today, a first-trimester abortion can be completed in 5 to 10 minutes, while a second-trimester procedure will take 15 to 45 minutes. Of course, every provider performs abortions a little differently, and specific surgical procedures may vary from clinic to clinic.

In the Examination Room

When it is time for your abortion, you will be taken to a special examination or procedure room and asked to undress from the waist down. You will be given a paper sheet or robe and left alone while you remove your clothes. The doctor and other clinic staff, such as a nurse or counselor, will enter the room once you have undressed. For the abortion, you will lie on an examination table with stirrups, or leg supports, and at some clinics, you may be able to see or hear the vacuum aspiration machine before or during the procedure.

At many clinics today, an abortion may be preceded by a pelvic examination. If you have never had a pelvic, or have not had one within the past year, the doctor will take a Pap smear—a test for cervical cancer—and do other tests to check for sexually transmitted diseases, such as chlamydia and gonorrhea. The doctor will also perform a "bimanual" or internal exam to determine the size and location of your uterus. For this part of the examination, the doctor will gently place two fingers in your vagina and his or her other hand on your abdomen.

To begin the abortion—or the pelvic if you are having one—a surgical instrument called a speculum will be inserted in your vagina. Made of either plastic or metal, the speculum is a duck-billed instrument that keeps the walls of your vagina apart and allows the doctor to see your cervix. Insertion and opening of the speculum may feel awkward and a little uncomfortable but should not cause any pain.

After the speculum is inserted, the walls of the vagina will be washed with an antiseptic to prevent infection, and if a local anesthetic is being used, it will be injected at this time. The injection—made directly to the cervix—feels like a pin prick. It may burn or hurt for a moment. Women using IV sedation or a general anesthetic can expect to receive a shot or be put on an IV drip right before the procedure; tranquilizers are usually given an hour or so ahead of time.

Vacuum Aspiration

The vacuum aspiration procedure is generally used for abortions during the first trimester (the first 12 to 14 weeks of pregnancy). At most clinics, you must be 6 to 7 weeks pregnant to have a vacuum aspiration, although some providers now perform the procedure at 3 to 5 weeks.

In the first part of the procedure, the cervix is made wider, or dilated, by the insertion of a series of very thin dilating rods. The rods are made of metal or plastic and are tapered at the end. Only a short section of the rod is inserted for dilation. The whole process takes only a minute or two.

For most first-trimester abortions, the first rod used is very narrow, about 2 millimeters wide, and the last one is about 8 millimeters, the size of a pencil or the tip of your little finger. If you are 12 to 14 weeks pregnant, you may need additional dilation; the last rod used may be slightly wider, 12 millimeters, or about the size of your thumb. If you are using a local anesthetic, dilation may cause some sharp, brief cramps, similar to what you might feel during a heavy period.

Once dilation is completed, a flexible, blunt-tipped plastic tube called a cannula is carefully and gently inserted into the uterus and then attached to a suction, or vacuum aspiration, machine. When the machine is turned on, you may hear a humming sound, and the contents of the uterus will be emptied. Additional cramping and physical discomfort may occur at this time, and women often say they feel as if something is pulling at their uterus. Near the end of the procedure, when the cannula is taken out of the vagina, you may also hear a sucking sound.

Note: At a few clinics, early abortions—before 5 weeks—are now being performed with a handheld syringe rather than a vacuum aspiration machine. These procedures are noiseless, and cramping and physical discomfort may be slightly less (see **Chapter 10**).

After the cannula is removed, many doctors gently scrape the walls of the uterus with a small, spoon-shaped instrument called a curette and then perform a quick, final suction. To ensure that the abortion is complete, extracted tissue is examined immediately after the procedure. If an incomplete abortion is suspected for any reason, you may be asked to return to the clinic in a day or two for an additional blood test or sonogram.

Dilation and Evacuation

Today, only half of all providers in the United States perform second-trimester abortions, and upper limits for the procedure vary widely. At some clinics, D & Es are only done up to the 16th or 18th week of pregnancy; at others, the limit is 20 or 22 weeks. Only a handful of providers go up to 24 or 25 weeks (see **Chapter 1**).

The main difference between vacuum aspiration and a D & E is the method of dilation. The cervix needs to be slightly wider for a second-trimester procedure because the fetus is larger. Laminaria, natural dilators made from sterile seaweed, are used to expand the cervix slowly and gently over a 1-to-2-day period. Some clinics also use synthetic dilators called Dilapan.

Dry laminaria are about the same size as kitchen matches. Once in the cervix, they absorb moisture and expand slowly, like a sponge. The number of laminaria used and the length of time required for dilation depend on the length of the pregnancy. For example, if you are 15 weeks pregnant, only a few laminaria will be used, but at 18 weeks you may need five or more. Laminaria are usually inserted the day before the abortion itself. Late in the second trimester, two or more insertions may be needed over a 2-day period.

Depending on the number of laminaria being used, insertion can take as little as 2 to 3 minutes or as long as 15 to 20 minutes. Sharp but brief cramping may occur at this time, and women may also experience less severe cramping and pain during the first few hours of dilation. At some clinics, a local anesthetic may be used for insertion, and your provider will tell you when and whether you should take pain medication such as acetaminophen (Tylenol) or ibuprofen for cramps. Laminaria are removed by the doctor just before the abortion. If the cervix still isn't dilated enough, the doctor may also use dilating rods similar to the ones used for a vacuum aspiration procedure.

Note: Once laminaria are inserted, you may be required to stay within a 30-to-60-minute drive of the clinic. You may also need a driver or other support person to stay with you to ensure you can call or get back to the clinic quickly if any complications develop. You will be given the clinic's 24-hour emergency number, and most providers will be able to refer you to a reasonably priced hotel in the area (see **Chapter 6**). If you change your mind, laminaria can be removed, and dilation stopped at any time before the abortion. However, stopping the procedure at this point may increase your risk for miscarriage, infection, and other complications.

Fetal Demise For abortions after the 18th or 19th week, some providers use an injection of a drug called digoxin or a similar medication to stop the fetal heartbeat and ensure fetal demise before the procedure. The injection usually occurs at the same time as laminaria insertion and is made directly to the uterus. *At this point, you will not be able to change your mind, and the abortion will have to be completed.*

Your preabortion counseling session should include full information on any drugs to be used for your abortion, and the counselor will answer any questions you may have at that time.

Evacuation   For second-trimester abortions, a combination of surgical instruments and procedures are used to empty the uterus. In most cases, the doctor will first use a vacuum aspiration machine to remove fluid and tissue. Additional fetal tissue is removed with forceps and curettes, and a final suction may be performed and fetal tissue examined to ensure that the abortion is complete.

An evacuation will take about 15 to 45 minutes, depending on how long you have been pregnant. The procedure can be done with a local anesthetic; however, IV sedation or general anesthetics are often available at clinics that perform D & Es. Depending on the anesthetic you choose, you can expect moderate to heavy cramping and physical discomfort during and after the procedure. Even if you've only had a local anesthetic, you may still need someone to drive you home from the clinic.

Pain and Cramping

When a pregnancy is terminated, the uterus contracts. The resulting cramps and abdominal pain are a normal part of the abortion procedure. For some women, abortion-related cramping will be no worse than what they feel during a regular menstrual period; others may experience brief but intense abdominal pain. IV sedation or a general anesthetic may reduce pain during the procedure, but you can still expect some cramps and physical discomfort afterward.

Any pain and cramping—and your risk for complications—are likely to increase if you tense up during the abortion. In particular, tensing the muscles in your thighs or abdomen can make it more difficult for a provider to complete the procedure quickly and safely.

Try to relax. Many clinics decorate the ceilings over their examination tables with travel posters so women have something pleasant, or at least distracting, to look at during the abortion. If you are blind or have any other visual disability, you can ask the clinic to play music, or you can bring a small CD or tape player and a favorite disk or cassette. Breathing from your stomach and taking deep breaths may also help, and a nurse or counselor will be in the room to hold your hand and talk with you throughout the procedure.

Note: Extremely sharp pain or cramping may be the first sign of a possible complication. If you experience any sudden, severe, or intolerable pain during the abortion, *tell the doctor immediately.* If sudden or heavy cramping occurs after you leave the clinic, *call your provider.*

Bleeding

Bleeding is also a normal side effect of abortion, and you can expect light to moderate bleeding after the procedure. Bleeding will usually last only a few days, but some women may bleed for a week to 10 days or longer. Use sanitary pads, not tampons, at this time.

Bleeding should be monitored carefully, especially during the first few hours and days after an abortion when heavy or abnormal bleeding may be the first sign of an incomplete procedure or other complications. Most clinics define heavy bleeding as bleeding through more than one extra-thick sanitary pad per hour for 2 to 3 hours. If this occurs, *call your provider immediately.*

AFTERCARE

After your abortion, you will stay at the clinic for a short time to recover from the procedure and receive postabortion counseling, including aftercare instructions and information on birth control. Most clinics have special recovery rooms furnished with comfortable reclining chairs or sofas. Women are given heating pads and light snacks, such as crackers, soda, and fruit juice. A nurse or specially trained counselor will check for any signs of complications, and you can stay in the room until you feel well enough to leave.

In general, if you have had a first-trimester abortion with a local anesthetic, your recovery time will be about 20 to 30 minutes. For second-trimester abortions or procedures done with additional pain medication, recovery times are usually longer: 30 minutes to an hour. In some cases, women who live more than 2 hours from the clinic may be kept in the recovery room for 2 hours or more to ensure that no complications develop before they go home (see **Chapter 6**).

While you are in the recovery room, a nurse or counselor will talk with you about aftercare. Many providers give women medication to prevent infection and stop heavy bleeding, or a prescription to fill at a local pharmacy. You will receive an information sheet detailing what physical activities to avoid for the next few days and weeks and how to monitor yourself

---

VIEWING FETAL TISSUE

After an abortion, some women want to see the tissue—what doctors call the "products of conception"—that has been removed from their bodies. Some providers now ask all women if they want to see fetal tissue, but at most clinics you will have to make a special request either when you make your appointment or during your preabortion counseling session.

Women have many reasons for wanting or not wanting to see fetal tissue, and at most clinics, women who ask to see the tissue are not judged or treated any differently from those who don't. Some women feel that viewing fetal tissue is grisly or just unnecessary and would never think to ask. For others, seeing the tissue is reassuring; it reconfirms their decision and provides a sense of closure or finality. Some women are simply curious; others consider viewing the tissue as a part of their personal grieving or recovery process.

If you decide to look at fetal tissue, you should be prepared mentally and emotionally for what you are going to see. At some clinics, you may be required to look at a booklet with pictures and detailed descriptions of fetal tissue or may receive additional counseling before and after the abortion. Viewing the tissue usually occurs in an examination or counseling room—somewhere private—and you can be left alone or have a partner, counselor, or other support person in the room with you.

---

for any signs of complications. Follow all aftercare instructions carefully, and call the clinic *immediately* if you develop a fever over 100.4 degrees or experience heavy bleeding or cramping (see **Bleeding,** p. 155). Most clinics have a 24-hour emergency line, and you should be sure that you have this number before you leave the clinic.

Birth control counseling and supplies are also available at most clinics. In many cases, you can begin using a new or different method almost immediately. At some clinics, women can receive Depo-Provera injections or Norplant insertions the same day as their procedure, and condoms, contraceptive foam, and birth control pills are often given to abortion patients free of charge. Your counselor will talk with you about the most effective ways to use birth control to prevent both unplanned pregnancies and sexually transmitted diseases. Information and supplies will also be available when you return from your follow-up appointment.

YOUR FOLLOW-UP APPOINTMENT

Y Most clinics recommend a follow-up appointment 2 to 3 weeks after an abortion to ensure that you are fully recovered from the procedure, physically and emotionally. You can schedule the appointment before you leave the clinic or call back in a few days' time. If you live in a different city or state and cannot return for a follow-up, ask for a referral to a pro-choice clinic or doctor in your area. At most clinics, the follow-up appointment is included in the cost of your abortion. If you go to a different provider, you will be charged an additional office fee.

However good you feel after an abortion, *don't skip your follow-up!* Hidden complications can develop, and a physical exam is necessary to make sure you are no longer pregnant and your recovery is complete.

Some women do feel sad, angry, or depressed for a few days or weeks after an abortion—this is normal; it does *not* mean you have "postabortion trauma syndrome"—and counseling is available at many clinics. Hour-long sessions are free and confidential and can be arranged at any time; you don't have to wait till your follow-up. In emergencies, a counselor will speak with you over the phone, and women seeking long-term counseling or other services can receive referrals to therapists, community health organizations, and local women's groups (see **Chapter 8**).

GETTING AN ABORTION:
AT A GLANCE

• Abortion is one of the safest and most common surgical procedures performed in the United States today. It does not cause sterility or breast cancer, and less than 1 percent of women who have abortions develop complications after the procedure.

• To find out how long you have been pregnant, count from the first day of your last normal period. If you are in the first trimester, the first 12 to 14 weeks, you will have a vacuum aspiration abortion. In the second trimester, between the 13th and 24th or 25th weeks, the procedure is called dilation and evacuation, or D & E.

• At most clinics, a first-trimester abortion can be done in one appointment. A second-trimester abortion may take two or three appointments.

• Write down any information or instructions you are given when you make your appointment. If you are having a second-trimester abortion or extra pain medication, you will not be allowed to drive after the procedure.

+ The abortion procedure is only part of the comprehensive care provided at most clinics. Your appointment will also include pregnancy and blood tests, a sonogram, counseling, and aftercare. Expect to be at the clinic for about 2 to 5 hours.

+ The first-trimester abortion procedure, vacuum aspiration, takes about 5 to 10 minutes and is usually done with a local anesthetic. Very small dilating rods are used to expand the cervix, and fetal tissue is removed with a vacuum aspiration machine and curettes.

+ D & Es are usually 2-to-3-day procedures. The cervix is slowly dilated with laminaria over a 1-to-2-day period. The abortion is performed on the second or third day and takes about 15 to 45 minutes. Fetal tissue is removed with vacuum aspiration, curettes, and forceps.

+ With a local anesthetic or tranquilizers, you will be conscious during the abortion and will feel some cramping and physical discomfort. With IV sedation or a general anesthetic, you will not remember the procedure, but you may experience cramps, dizziness, and other side effects afterward.

+ To minimize cramps during an abortion, try to relax. Breathe from your stomach, take deep breaths, and try not to tense your thighs or stomach. If you experience any sudden, unusual, or intolerable pain, *tell the doctor immediately.*

+ After the abortion, you will stay in a special recovery room for 20 minutes to an hour and receive information on aftercare and birth control. You will also get a 24-hour emergency number. Call immediately if you develop a fever of 100.4 degrees or more or experience heavy cramps or bleeding.

+ A follow-up appointment 2 to 3 weeks after the abortion is *essential* to make sure you are fully recovered, physically and emotionally. If you live in another city or state, ask for a referral to a prochoice clinic or doctor in your area.

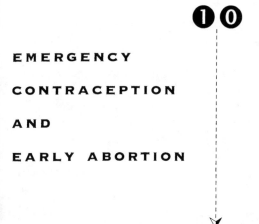

EMERGENCY CONTRACEPTION AND EARLY ABORTION

Read this chapter if you have had unprotected sex within the last 2 or 3 days and don't want to get pregnant; or if you are less than 6 or 7 weeks pregnant and don't want to wait to have an abortion.

For many women, the hardest part of any unplanned pregnancy is waiting. Waiting to find out if you are pregnant after the condom breaks or a sudden, impulsive act of unprotected sex—yes, it happens, even to women who are usually very careful about birth control. Waiting more, 1 to 3 weeks, because you're less than 6 or 7 weeks pregnant and your provider won't perform a vacuum aspiration before then, no matter how quickly you call the clinic and have a test.

Fortunately, for a growing number of women, waiting—and all the worry and stress it can cause—may no longer be necessary. With recent advances in reproductive health care, women now have more options for stopping a pregnancy in the first few days after unprotected sex and getting an abortion very early in the first trimester, in some cases even before you miss a period.

Studies show that emergency contraception, or "morning-after pills," taken within 48 to 72 hours of unprotected sex can prevent unplanned pregnancies in at least 75 percent of all cases. In addition, highly sensitive blood and urine tests now allow women to find out if they are pregnant as early as 10 days after conception, and some clinics will perform vacuum aspiration abortions at 3 to 5 weeks, instead of the usual 6 to 7.

Medical abortion—using the new abortion-inducing drugs mifepristone and methotrexate—is also available at a small but growing number of clinics. These drugs allow women to terminate pregnancies very early in the first trimester—up to the 7th or 8th week—without surgery and, in some but not all cases, in the privacy of their own homes.

While emergency contraception and medical abortion are often touted as quick, easy solutions to the problem of unplanned pregnancy, the potential of these new treatments must be balanced with their limitations. Emergency contraception is *not* a substitute for regular birth control, and medical abortion is unlikely to replace surgical abortion or put clinics— or unfortunately, antichoice protesters—out of business. At present, the availability of both treatments remains limited, and practical considerations—such as time, cost, and confidentiality—may mean they will not be accessible or appropriate for all women (see **Medical Abortion versus Vacuum Aspiration**, p. 170).

This chapter provides basic information on emergency contraception and early abortion and some of their advantages and drawbacks. The topics covered include:

+ Emergency contraception and how to find a clinic or family planning center where you can get it

+ Why providers can now perform vacuum aspiration abortions before the 6th or 7th week of pregnancy

+ Medical abortion, what it's like, and the differences between mifepristone and methotrexate

+ Medical versus surgical abortion—how they compare

EMERGENCY CONTRACEPTION

Emergency contraceptive pills are high doses of regular birth control pills taken within the first 48 to 72 hours after contraceptive failure or other unprotected sex. Only certain brands of pills can be used, and a prescription from a licensed physician is needed to get them. This means you must call a doctor or clinic first. *Do not use birth control pills a friend gives you or an old prescription you find in a drawer or medicine cabinet at home.*

How do the pills work? Researchers don't know exactly, but believe that when taken in high doses, the hormones in birth control pills interfere with a woman's normal hormonal patterns and make it impossible for a fertilized egg to become attached, or implanted, to the wall of the uterus. Implantation usually takes place the 5th or 6th day after conception, and most doctors do not consider a woman to be pregnant until this occurs.

After implantation, emergency contraception will not work. *Time is criti-cal.* Any woman who has had unprotected sex and does not want to be-come pregnant should contact a clinic or other emergency contraception provider immediately.

How to Find Emergency Contraception

To find a clinic or other emergency contraception provider near you, call the **Emergency Contraception Hotline.** Referrals are also available on the World Wide Web at the **Emergency Contraception Home Page.**

* Emergency Contraception Hotline   800-584-9911

* Emergency Contraception Home Page   http://opr.princeton.edu/ec/

The Emergency Contraception Hotline provides recorded information on emergency contraception and referrals to local clinics and doctors who offer the pills. The line is open 24 hours a day, 7 days a week, and all calls are free and confidential. The Emergency Contraception Home Page contains similar information and a constantly updated provider referral list. Providers include prochoice clinics, family planning centers, public health centers, university student health clinics, and private doctors.

Note: In some instances, university clinics may only provide services to students and school employees. In addition, while most clinics offering emergency contraception will schedule an appointment for you on an im-mediate, drop-in basis, delays can occur, and you could be told that you will not be able to get an appointment for several days or longer. To avoid any scheduling problems, be sure to tell the phone counselor or other clinic staff that you have had unprotected sex and need to make an ap-pointment for emergency contraception. If an appointment cannot be scheduled within 48 to 72 hours, *don't give up!* Check the Emergency Contraception Hotline or Home Page, and call another clinic or provider in your area.

What to Expect

While some providers will arrange a prescription for emergency contra-ception over the phone, others may require you to come in for an ap-pointment. Costs vary widely and may *not* be covered by Medicaid or private insurance. Even if you can get a prescription over the phone, you can expect to pay as much as $30 to $35 for the pills. Appointment fees can range from $40 to over $100.

If an appointment is necessary, it should take an hour or less. You will fill out a medical history form, and a counselor will give you information on emergency contraception, how and when to take the pills, and possible side effects. You will be asked for the first day of your last normal menstrual period, when you had unprotected sex, and whether you need information on birth control. A physical exam and pelvic may also be performed.

In some cases, emergency contraception is not recommended for women who are over 40 and heavy smokers or for women with any of the following medical conditions:

- Blood clots in veins

- Liver disease

- Inflammation of the veins

- Unexplained vaginal bleeding

- Any suspicion of breast cancer or any other cancer of the reproductive organs, such as cervical, ovarian, or uterine cancer

Women with these disorders may still be able to take the pills but should check with a counselor or doctor first.

In general, two kinds of birth control pills are used for emergency contraception—combined and mini. If your provider uses combined pills, which contain both estrogen and progesterone, you will be given either 4 or 8 pills: half to be taken at the clinic and half to be taken 12 hours later. Minipills only contain progesterone and are used for women who cannot take estrogen. The dosage is much higher: 20 pills at the clinic and 20 more 12 hours later. Combined pills can be taken up to 72 hours after unprotected sex; minipills must be taken within 48 hours.

Taking the pills may cause some physical discomfort, including nausea, vomiting, breast tenderness, abdominal pain, and headaches. These side effects usually last 1 to 2 days. Nausea and vomiting can often be controlled with Dramamine or other nonprescription drugs. If vomiting occurs within 2 hours of taking emergency contraception, you may need to call your provider or return to the clinic for additional pills.

Note: Recent studies indicate that nausea and vomiting can be reduced if emergency contraceptive pills are inserted in the vagina, rather than taken orally. If your first dose of pills causes vomiting, ask your provider about trying vaginal insertion for the second dose.

You will not know if the emergency contraception has worked until you get your period, which should occur in 2 to 3 weeks. If you do not get your period, or have only light or abnormal spotting, call your clinic or family planning center and arrange for a pregnancy test.

INTRAUTERINE DEVICES

Another method of birth control called an intrauterine device, or IUD, can also be used as emergency contraception. At present, the IUD available at most clinics is a small, plastic, T-shaped device called a Copper-T, that is inserted in the uterus. To prevent an unplanned pregnancy, insertion must occur within 5 to 7 days of contraceptive failure or unprotected sex. Studies show that IUDs used as emergency contraception are 99 percent effective; however, they are often recommended only for women who intend to use them as their regular form of birth control. Information on IUDs is available at most clinics and family planning centers.

EARLY SURGICAL ABORTION

Until recently, no matter how early a woman called a clinic for a pregnancy test and counseling, she would usually be told that an abortion could not be performed until she was 6 or 7 weeks pregnant. Before 6 weeks, the pregnancy was considered too small, and most providers were concerned about an increased risk of incomplete or missed abortion or other complications.

While previously valid, providers' attitudes and fears about early abortion have now begun to change. Again, highly sensitive blood and urine tests can diagnose a pregnancy 10 days after conception, and a vacuum aspiration can be performed as soon as the pregnancy is visible on a sonogram, which, with advanced ultrasound equipment, is now possible at 4 to 5 weeks. Availability remains limited, but a small number of clinics are beginning to offer early vacuum aspiration.

Having a surgical abortion at 4 to 5 weeks is essentially no different than having one at any time during the first trimester and, at most clinics, it will cost about the same. The cervix is dilated gently and carefully with very narrow dilating rods, and a vacuum aspiration machine or a hand-held suction pump is used to empty the uterus (see **The Handheld Pump**, below). The procedure takes 5 to 10 minutes or less and can be done with a local anesthetic. Cramping or physical discomfort may occur, but it will be minimal and brief.

In most cases, fetal tissue and other contents of the uterus are examined carefully after the procedure to ensure that the abortion is complete. If any signs of an incomplete or failed procedure are found, you may be required to return to the clinic in a day or two for an additional blood test or ultrasound.

THE HANDHELD PUMP

Vacuum aspiration performed with a handheld suction pump is a new and promising procedure for early abortion developed by Dr. Jerry Edwards of Planned Parenthood in Houston, Texas. It is similar to, but substantially different from menstrual extraction, a method for early abortion pioneered in the 1970s by women's health activists Carol Downer and Lorraine Rothman and still used by self-help groups of women who teach each other the procedure (see A Woman's Book of Choices, **Appendix 2**). For example, a menstrual extraction can take 15 minutes to a half-hour to complete, compared to 5 minutes or less for early vacuum aspiration. Dr. Edwards also notes that the handheld pump may make the procedure less physically and emotionally stressful for some women. There is no suction or machine noise during the abortion, and cramping or other physical discomfort may also be reduced.

In addition, procedures done with a handheld pump can be performed as early as 3 weeks—even before a pregnancy is visible on a sonogram. In such instances, an extra blood test is required after the procedure, and tissue is carefully examined to make sure the abortion is complete. An incomplete or unsuccessful abortion at this time could be the first sign of an ectopic, or tubal, pregnancy—a potentially dangerous condition where the fertilized egg becomes implanted in the fallopian tube rather than the uterus. *An ectopic pregnancy can cause permanent damage to the fallopian tubes and must be terminated as quickly as possible.* If an ectopic pregnancy is suspected, you will be referred to a hospital for additional tests and treatment. When diagnosed early in the first trimester, an ectopic pregnancy can be quickly and safely terminated with methotrexate, and in most cases, surgery will not be required.

MIFEPRISTONE AND METHOTREXATE: A COMPARISON

	Mifepristone (RU-486)	Methotrexate
How it works	Antiprogesterone: blocks implantation of fertilized egg in uterus	Antimetabolite: stops growth of fetus
When to use	FDA expected to approve for use up to the 7th week of pregnancy; can be used up to the 8th or 9th	Up to the 7th or 8th week of pregnancy
Effectiveness	95 to 97% up to the 7th week; in the 8th or 9th week, increased chance of delayed or failed abortion	90 to 95%
Treatment protocol	3 pills taken orally, followed by misoprostol, orally or as vaginal insertion 36 to 48 hours later	Injection, amount depends on height and weight, followed by misoprostol as vaginal insertion 5 to 7 days later
Appointments	If misoprostol is taken at the clinic, 2; if taken at home, 1	Same
Side effects	Heavy cramping and bleeding; misoprostol may cause chills, fever, dizziness, diarrhea, headaches, nausea, and vomiting; side effects stop when abortion is complete	Same; side effects of misoprostol may be less severe
How long it takes	76% of women will expel within 2 to 24 hours after taking misoprostol; others may need additional misoprostol or vacuum aspiration	50 to 60% of women will expel within 2 to 24 hours; others may need additional misoprostol or vacuum aspiration; delays of 4 to 6 weeks occur in 5 to 10 percent of all cases
Birth defects	Mifepristone does not cause birth defects, but misoprostol does. If abortion is delayed or not successful, a surgical procedure is required	Causes birth defects; if abortion is delayed or not successful, a surgical procedure is required
Postabortion bleeding and spotting	A few days to 2 to 4 weeks	Same

MEDICAL ABORTION

✔ **Medical abortion** is the term most providers now use to refer to the abortion-inducing drugs mifepristone (RU-486) and methotrexate. These drugs can be used to terminate a pregnancy at any time during the first 7 to 8 weeks of pregnancy, measured from the first day of a woman's last normal menstrual period. You do not have to wait to call or go to the clinic.

If your provider offers medical abortion, you will be screened to make sure the drugs are safe for you to use. A positive pregnancy test will be required, and the clinic may also perform a sonogram to confirm that your pregnancy is not too far advanced. Your preabortion counseling will include full information on the drugs you are using and their possible side effects. You will also have to comply with any informed consent or parental involvement laws in your state.

Whether you use mifepristone or methotrexate—the drugs work in slightly different ways (see **Mifepristone and Methotrexate: A Comparison**, p. 165)—the abortion itself will be a two-step procedure. Women first receive pills (mifepristone) or a shot (methotrexate) to interrupt or stop fetal development. The abortion is completed 2 to 7 days later with a second drug, misoprostol, that causes the uterus to contract and expel the pregnancy. Women using mifepristone may have to return to the clinic for the misoprostol; with methotrexate, the misoprostol can often be taken at home. Expulsion usually occurs within 2 to 24 hours; however, it can be delayed several days or weeks. In such cases, additional doses of misoprostol may be required or a vacuum aspiration can be performed.

Any provider who offers medical abortion should be able to perform vacuum aspiration or refer you to a nearby doctor, clinic, or hospital that does. This is essential to ensure that a surgical abortion can be performed if the medical procedure is not successful or complications develop (see **Bleeding, Cramping, . . . ,** p. 169). Some providers may also require that you live within 2 hours of the clinic or a medical facility, like a hospital, where emergency care is available.

If you go to a provider that does not perform vacuum aspiration, and a surgical procedure becomes necessary, it will probably *not* be included in the cost of your abortion, and you will have to pay an additional fee to the doctor or clinic you are referred to. Most providers charge $300 to $450 for vacuum aspiration, and an emergency abortion at a hospital can cost between $500 and $1,000.

In addition, although current studies indicate that mifepristone does not cause birth defects, both methotrexate and misoprostol do. This means that if a medical abortion is not successful, you should *not* continue the pregnancy, and a surgical procedure will be necessary.

Research and government regulations on the use and availability of mifepristone and methotrexate are continuing to change, and medical protocols may vary from provider to provider. Your doctor or clinic will be able to answer any questions you have on the safety and effectiveness of medical abortion and the specific drugs they use.

Mifepristone

Mifepristone (RU-486) was developed in the 1970s in France, where it is now used for about one-third of all abortions. It has also been tested and used successfully in Britain, Sweden, China, and, most recently, the United States. Once approved by the Food and Drug Administration (FDA), it will be available from clinics and licensed physicians.

Mifepristone works by blocking a hormone called progesterone, which is essential to maintaining a pregnancy in its early stages. If progesterone is blocked, the fertilized egg or embryo cannot attach itself to the wall of the uterus. The drug also makes the uterus softer and more sensitive to misoprostol, so expulsion occurs quickly when the second drug is taken, usually 2 days later.

Mifepristone is not recommended for women who are over 35 and smoke more than 10 cigarettes a day. The drug may also not be safe for women with any of the following medical conditions:

- Uncontrolled or untreated hypertension or high blood pressure

- Diabetes

- Ovarian masses—but not cysts—or other reproductive tumors

- Severe asthma

- Severe anemia

A medical abortion with mifepristone may require two appointments: one to get counseling and the pills—the usual dose is three pills—and the second, 2 days later, for the misoprostol, which may be taken orally or as a vaginal insertion. Expulsion usually occurs within 2 to 4 hours, and your provider may require you to remain at the clinic during this time.

Note: FDA guidelines for mifepristone recommend women stay at the clinic after taking misoprostol, but this may not be necessary. Recent studies indicate that misoprostol can be taken safely at home with mifepristone as well as methotrexate.

Mifepristone is about 95 to 97 percent effective during the first 7 weeks of pregnancies. The drug can be used up to the 8th or 9th week; however, the risk of a delayed or incomplete abortion increases, and additional doses of misoprostol or a vacuum aspiration may be needed to complete the procedure (see **Delayed Abortion,** p. 170).

Methotrexate

Methotrexate has been legal in the United States since 1954, when it was approved for the treatment of cancer, psoriasis, and arthritis. In 1982, doctors began using it to terminate ectopic, or tubal, pregnancies, and more recently, it has been used for medical abortions up to the 7th or 8th week of pregnancy. Availability is still limited, but a growing number of providers are now offering methotrexate as an early-abortion option.

Methotrexate works by blocking a specific vitamin, folic acid, that is necessary for cell division. Once you take the drug, the fetus stops growing. Methotrexate is toxic, but studies seem to indicate that the relatively small amount used for early abortion is safe for most women. It is not recommended if you have severe anemia or severe liver or kidney disease.

Methotrexate is slightly more complicated to use than mifepristone. The drug is injected—you get a shot—and the amount used will depend on your height and weight. You may be told not to have sex until the abortion is complete. Some providers will also tell you not to take vitamins or eat foods with folic acid, such as leafy green vegetables, whole grains, oranges, and grapefruit.

To complete the abortion, misoprostol is inserted into the vagina about 5 to 7 days later, either at the clinic or by the woman herself at home. Women taking misoprostol at home will be given detailed information on when and how to insert the pills and what to expect when expulsion occurs.

While methotrexate is 90 to 95 percent effective, expulsion of the pregnancy can be delayed and unpredictable. In most cases—50 to 60 percent—the abortion will be complete within 2 to 24 hours, but some women may have to wait several days or weeks. An additional dose of misoprostol or a vacuum aspiration may then be required (see **Delayed Abortion,** p. 170).

Note: Although methotrexate stops fetal growth, it may *not* stop some symptoms of pregnancy. Pregnancy symptoms like morning sickness and breast tenderness may continue until the abortion is complete.

Bleeding, Cramping, and Other Side Effects

Medical abortion with mifepristone or methotrexate is often compared to a miscarriage. After taking the misoprostol, women may experience heavy cramping and bleeding, and large clots of tissue may be expelled. Misoprostol may also cause other side effects, including chills, headaches, dizziness, fever, diarrhea, nausea, and vomiting.

The experience of individual women will vary, depending on whether they are using mifepristone or methotrexate and how the drugs affect them. In one study on methotrexate, two-thirds of the women experienced nausea after taking the misoprostol, while in another, only 11 percent did. In U.S. tests on mifepristone, half the women said the procedure was less painful than they had expected, and only 20 percent needed medication to control cramping and other physical discomfort.

In general, providers report that with mifepristone, the onset of side effects occurs relatively quickly and dramatically once the misoprostol is taken. In particular, chills and cramping may begin within 20 or 30 minutes. With methotrexate, side effects are less intense and may take longer to begin. Most clinics provide acetaminophen (Tylenol) with codeine for women who experience heavy cramping or other physical discomforts, and symptoms stop almost immediately when the abortion is complete. Postabortion bleeding and spotting is also common and may continue for several days or up to 2 to 4 weeks.

Note: Severity of side effects may also depend on whether misoprostol is taken orally or as a vaginal insertion. Recent studies seem to indicate that with insertion, headaches, diarrhea, nausea, and other symptoms are less acute.

Heavy clotting and bleeding is a *normal* part of any medical abortion. Once expulsion begins, you can expect to make repeated trips to the bathroom for 2 to 4 hours, and you may pass very large clots. According to Dr. Suzanne Poppema of Seattle, Washington, clots "the size of an orange or grapefruit" are not uncommon.

If you are taking misoprostol at home, you will have to monitor bleeding and other side effects carefully and follow any instructions you receive at the clinic. Your provider will also give you a 24-hour number to call in case of complications, such as uncontrolled bleeding or cramping. As with surgical abortion, if you are bleeding through more than one extrathick sanitary pad per hour for more than 2 or 3 hours, *call the clinic immediately.* Uncontrolled bleeding could be a sign of an incomplete abortion, and you may need to return to the clinic for a surgical procedure.

MEDICAL ABORTION VERSUS VACUUM ASPIRATION

Is medical abortion the magic pill that, as some prochoice providers and activists have claimed, will allow women to be in complete control of their abortions and make clinic harassment a thing of the past? At this point, it is impossible to say how mifepristone and methotrexate will affect women's access to abortion: whether private or family doctors will offer the drugs, how antichoice groups will react, or if women will come to prefer medical abortion to vacuum aspiration.

DELAYED ABORTION

Studies show that 3 to 10 percent of all women taking mifepristone and methotrexate can expect a delayed or unsuccessful abortion. Delays of 4 to 5 weeks are rare, but not abnormal, especially with methotrexate. A delayed abortion does **not** mean that you are still pregnant. Both mifepristone and methotrexate interrupt fetal development, and fetal growth and heartbeat should stop shortly after you take the drugs.

In most cases, if expulsion does not occur within 3 to 7 days, you will return to the clinic for additional medical tests and a second dose of misoprostol. Depending on your provider, further delays may be treated with more misoprostol or a surgical abortion. You can also ask for a surgical abortion at any time if you are anxious about a delayed expulsion or don't want to take additional misoprostol.

A medical abortion is considered unsuccessful if expulsion has not occurred within 5 or 6 weeks or if any signs of ongoing fetal development are discovered. In such cases, a vacuum aspiration procedure will be performed.

What can be said right now is that the drugs are safe, and they will provide some women with additional options for terminating unplanned pregnancies. Current studies show that about one-third of all women seeking abortions are less than 7 to 8 weeks pregnant, and the procedure they choose—medical or surgical—usually depends on a range of factors.

A woman who feels that any surgical procedure is intrusive or "unnatural" may be more comfortable with a medical abortion, while vacuum aspiration will be more practical if you want to avoid extra appointments or an unpredictable expulsion. Other considerations may include the safety and effectiveness of the two procedures, their cost, concerns about physical discomfort and bleeding, and which procedure will provide the most confidentiality.

Safety and Effectiveness

The safety and effectiveness of medical and surgical abortion are comparable. Vacuum aspiration is more effective—99 percent—compared to 95 to 97 percent for mifepristone and 90 to 95 percent for methotrexate. This means that 3 to 10 percent of all women taking mifepristone or methotrexate will have an incomplete or failed abortion and will need to return to their clinic for a surgical procedure.

With vacuum aspiration, the need for repeat surgery, or resuction, is only about 1 percent. On the other hand, the procedure is more intrusive—surgical instruments are used—and postabortion complications, such as infection and perforation of the uterus, are potentially more serious. However, the risk of complications is extremely low—less than 1 percent—and hospitalization is required in fewer than 1 in 200 cases.

Time and Money

How much an abortion costs and how long it takes are critical considerations for many women. Here, again, vacuum aspiration may be a slightly more practical choice. A surgical abortion can be completed in one 3-to-5-hour appointment, compared to the 2-step procedure and 2 to 7 days required for mifepristone and methotrexate.

Women taking mifepristone may need to make two appointments and stay at the clinic for 2 to 4 hours after taking the misoprostol. According to providers, preabortion counseling sessions for medical abortion may also take longer because women must receive detailed information on the side effects of misoprostol and what to expect when the pregnancy is expelled.

Additional appointments may also be necessary if expulsion is delayed and a second dose of misoprostol or a vacuum aspiration is required.

At present, most providers are charging the same for both medical and surgical abortions, around $300 to $450. Prices for medical abortion may increase, however, because of the extra appointments, medical tests, and time at the clinic the procedure requires. You may also have to pay extra if you have a delayed or unsuccessful abortion and must be referred to another doctor or clinic for vacuum aspiration (see **Medical Abortion**, p. 166).

Confidentiality

Which procedure—medical or surgical—can better safeguard women's confidentiality is an open question that depends largely on personal circumstances. At present, medical abortion is available primarily at clinics that offer vacuum aspiration, and that may mean taking time off, coming up with excuses, or being exposed to antichoice harassment (see **Chapter 7**). Similarly, being able to take misoprostol at home is no guarantee of confidentiality. Again, onset of expulsion and heavy cramping and bleeding may be unpredictable and raise the suspicions of partners, parents, or other friends and family members. Some women may feel safer or more comfortable taking misoprostol at a clinic or having a support person with them if they take it at home.

Cramping, Bleeding, and Aftercare

Any woman terminating an unplanned pregnancy can expect to experience some pain and cramping during the procedure and bleeding for several days afterward. With surgical abortion, the pain is usually described as minimal and brief—like heavy menstrual cramps—and women who use a local anesthetic are able to leave the clinic 20 to 30 minutes after the procedure. Women using IV sedation or a general anesthetic usually experience no pain during the procedure, but some cramping may occur after the medication wears off, and recovery time at the clinic may be an hour or longer. General anesthetics may also cause some side effects, such as headaches, dizziness, nausea, and vomiting. Bleeding during and immediately after the procedure is also minimal, and postabortion spotting usually lasts no longer than a week to 10 days.

Pain during a medical abortion has also been compared to heavy menstrual cramps; however, the physical discomfort usually lasts longer—an hour or more—and side effects from the misoprostol may include chills, fever, dizziness, headaches, diarrhea, nausea, and vomiting. Bleeding is heavier as well—again, you can expect to pass very large clots of tissue—and postabortion spotting may last longer, up to 2 to 4 weeks.

Aftercare for surgical and medical abortion is similar. Women who take mifepristone or methotrexate may not have to take antibiotics, but you will have to monitor yourself for signs of infection and other complications. A follow-up appointment will also be required 2 to 3 weeks after the abortion (see **Chapter 9**).

What Women Say

How do women feel about medical abortion? In recent studies on mifepristone and methotrexate, women have said they were satisfied with the drugs and would recommend them to others. Most women said that medical abortion was more "natural" and less intrusive or frightening than a surgical procedure, and they felt more in control of their treatment.

For some women, however, the emotional appeal of medical abortion is often balanced by more personal and practical considerations. In one recent study where women under 7 weeks pregnant were given information on both vacuum aspiration and methotrexate, 75 percent chose vacuum aspiration because, they said, they "just wanted to get the abortion over with" as quickly as possible. Other reasons for choosing the surgical procedure included fewer appointments and concerns about confidentiality if expulsion occurred at home. In another study, only 18 percent of women given information on medical abortion said they would choose the procedure; 40 percent said they would not, and 42 percent were undecided.

EMERGENCY CONTRACEPTION AND EARLY ABORTION: AT A GLANCE

- If the condom breaks, ***don't wait!*** Emergency contraceptives, or "morning-after" pills, are 75 percent effective in preventing unplanned pregnancy if taken within 2 to 3 days of unprotected sex.

- You ***must*** call a clinic to get emergency contraception. Referrals are available from the Emergency Contraception Hotline at 800-584-9911 and the Emergency Contraception Home Page at http://opr.princeton.edu/ec/.

- If you think you might be pregnant, don't wait until you miss a period to get a test. Most clinics now offer tests that can diagnose pregnancy as early as 10 days after conception.

+ Surgical abortion is now available at some clinics even if you are less than 6 or 7 weeks pregnant. The procedure is the same as a regular first-trimester procedure, and just as safe.

+ Medical abortion is the term most providers now use to refer to the abortion-inducing drugs mifepristone (RU-486) and methotrexate. The drugs can be used at any time during the first 7 or 8 weeks of pregnancy and cost about the same as a surgical abortion.

+ Medical abortion is usually a two-step procedure. You receive pills (mifepristone) or a shot (methotrexate). After 2 to 7 days, you take a second drug called misoprostol which causes the uterus to contract and expel the pregnancy.

+ Mifepristone interrupts pregnancy by blocking implantation of the embryo in the uterus. If you take mifepristone, you may be required to take the misoprostol at the clinic and remain there for 2 to 4 hours until the abortion is complete.

+ Methotrexate works by stopping cell division and fetal growth. With methotrexate, misoprostol can be taken at home, but expulsion may be unpredictable or delayed several days or weeks.

+ Medical abortion is similar to a miscarriage. You will experience heavy cramping and bleeding and may pass large clots of tissue. Misoprostol may also cause side effects, such as chills, headaches, fever, dizziness, diarrhea, and nausea.

+ If expulsion is delayed more than 3 to 7 days, you may have to return to the clinic for a second dose of misoprostol. Further delays may be treated with additional misoprostol or a surgical procedure. You can also ask for a vacuum aspiration at any time.

+ Between 3 and 10 percent of all women who take mifepristone or methotrexate will have a delayed or failed abortion and need a surgical procedure. With vacuum aspiration, only 1 percent will have an incomplete abortion and need resuctioning.

+ Some women prefer medical abortion because it is less intrusive and more "natural" than vacuum aspiration. Others continue to choose surgical abortion for practical reasons, such as time, effectiveness, and concerns about confidentiality and physical discomfort.

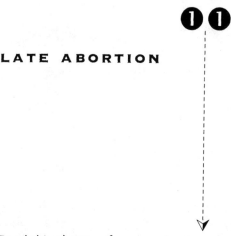

LATE ABORTION

Read this chapter if you are having an abortion in the second or third trimester because of a fetal anomaly or other life-threatening medical condition.

In most states today, abortion is illegal once the fetus becomes viable—is able to survive outside the womb—except in cases where a fetal anomaly, or defect, has been diagnosed or where carrying the pregnancy to term could put a woman's life at risk. The exact point of viability varies from pregnancy to pregnancy but usually occurs between the 24th and 28th weeks.

According to the National Abortion Federation, late, or third-trimester, abortions now account for less than 1 percent of all pregnancies terminated in the United States—about 600 per year. These procedures are often performed under heartbreaking, personally devastating circumstances and after careful consultation with doctors and other medical specialists. Only a small number of doctors and clinics perform late abortions, and most have special training and expertise in handling these cases.

This chapter contains a brief, basic overview of late abortion and some of the practical and emotional concerns you and your partner may face if terminating—or as some doctors say, interrupting—your pregnancy becomes necessary. It is *not* intended to be comprehensive, and you should expect to receive full information and counseling from your obstetrician and abortion provider. The topics covered here include:

* How and when fetal anomalies are diagnosed and why you shouldn't blame yourself for the baby's deformities

+ Finding providers that perform late abortions and some of the special services they may offer

+ Late abortion procedures and what doctors do to ensure they are safe and humane

+ Grieving and getting support after a late abortion

DIAGNOSIS AND COUNSELING

Fetal anomalies occur in 1 to 2 percent of all pregnancies. In many cases, they are *not* caused by genetic factors or anything a couple did or didn't do before or during a pregnancy. Defects just happen, and after an abortion, many women are able to get pregnant again and have healthy, normal children.

Unfortunately, even with early testing, diagnosis of anomalies may not occur until the second trimester of pregnancy, or even the third. Chorionic villus sampling—which involves taking a small sample of embryonic cells—can be performed as early as 10 to 13 weeks, but you won't receive results for 7 to 10 days. Amniocentesis, the most common test for defects, takes even longer. Fluid from the amniotic sac is drawn between the 16th and 18th week of pregnancy, and complete results are not available for 2 to 5 weeks. Ultrasound scans can also be used to diagnose defects, but if a pregnancy appears normal, only a few, routine scans may be performed, and an abnormality could be missed or not discovered until the 7th or 8th month.

When a defect is found or suspected, additional tests may be performed, and you and your partner will be referred to doctors and geneticists with special expertise in the fields of fetal development and defects. Once a specific abnormality has been diagnosed, you will receive counseling on the fetus's chances for survival and the kinds of treatment or ongoing care it might need if born alive. You will also be given information on terminating the pregnancy—if that is what you decide to do—and referrals to clinics or other providers who perform late abortions.

Note: Additional information on certain defects, such as Down syndrome and spina bifida, may be available from local or national organizations that provide support to families with children who have these disabilities. For example, before deciding to continue or terminate your pregnancy, you may be able to talk with parents who are raising a child with the same defect or disability as yours. Ask your doctor or clinic for referrals to specific groups. If a defect is genetic—such as Tay-Sachs disease—you will also need to talk with a doctor or counselor about whether future pregnancies should be considered.

The diagnosis of a fetal anomaly often leaves pregnant women and their partners feeling stunned, depressed, confused, and isolated. Women may feel guilty or think the defect was caused by something they did, or shouldn't have done—for example, drinking a few beers before they knew they were pregnant. The decision to terminate can be especially difficult if you and your partner are personally opposed to abortion or have previously been unable to get pregnant.

Talking about your feelings at this time can be essential. Many couples seek support from their doctors, clergy, or a few close friends and family members. Nonjudgmental, confidential counseling is also available at most clinics, and your provider may be able to refer you to therapists and support groups in your area (**Grieving and Getting Support**, p. 181).

FINDING A CLINIC

V If a late abortion becomes necessary, your doctor will probably refer you to the provider nearest you. Referrals are also available from the National Abortion Federation: in the United States, call 800-772-9100 and in Canada, call 800-424-2280.

Only a few doctors and clinics perform late abortions, and finding a provider can be difficult for emotional as well as practical reasons. Women and their partners may feel abandoned and upset when they are told that their obstetrician or regular gynecologist will not perform the procedure. Getting to the nearest provider may mean a long, emotionally draining trip to a clinic in another city or state. The need to make decisions quickly may also leave couples feeling numb or unable to ask for extra information or services.

While many women are, understandably, anxious to get a late abortion "over with" as quickly as possible, it is also important to take the time to think about what you and your partner may need from a provider—practically as well as emotionally—and *ask for it.* Clinics that perform late abortions frequently offer special services. Even small details can make a significant difference in what a couple feels and remembers about the experience. If you don't want to sit in a waiting room with other patients—especially women terminating unplanned but otherwise healthy pregnancies—ask for a private room. Many clinics will also allow your partner to stay with you throughout the procedure, and you can ask to see the fetus before you leave the clinic or arrange to have the body cremated or buried (see **Seeing the Fetus or Fetal Remains**, p. 180).

LATE-ABORTION PROCEDURES

In recent years, the topic of late abortion has become increasingly controversial and confusing. Efforts to outlaw the procedure, called intact dilation and extraction (IDE)—or "partial birth" abortion—have raised questions about the surgical methods doctors use in these cases and the safest, most humane way to terminate a pregnancy in the third trimester.

To begin with, the term *"partial birth" abortion* and antichoice claims that the procedure is inhumane are medically incorrect. Women who have late abortions are often given drugs to stop fetal heartbeat, and *the fetus is not alive at the time of the procedure.* The method chosen to terminate your pregnancy will depend on how long you have been pregnant and the specific surgical procedures your provider uses. The few doctors who perform late abortions employ similar, but slightly different methods. The procedure used will be the one that the doctor thinks least likely to damage a woman's cervix or affect her ability to carry future pregnancies to term.

INFORMED CONSENT LAWS

If your provider is located in a state with an informed consent law, find out if you have to comply with the law or if a waiver can be arranged. In some but not all cases, a late abortion for fetal anomalies is considered an emergency, and state-mandated lectures and waiting periods are not required.

Whenever possible, try to get a waiver. State-mandated materials often contain biased or misleading information and can be particularly upsetting for women terminating a wanted pregnancy. For example, you may be told that you could be eligible for medical benefits or welfare if you decide to continue the pregnancy or that having an abortion will increase your risk for breast cancer (see **Chapter 2**).

To get a waiver, you will need a special form or letter signed either by the doctor who performs your abortion or another licensed physician. Your provider will be able to tell you about the law in your state and how to arrange a waiver.

For abortions before 24 to 25 weeks, most clinics perform a regular dilation and evacuation (D & E). The cervix is dilated gradually with laminaria over a period of 1 to 2 days, and the pregnancy is removed with vacuum aspiration, forceps, and curettage. Depending on length of pregnancy, the procedure takes 15 to 45 minutes and can be done with a local anesthetic, IV sedation, or general anesthetic (see **Chapter 9**).

Abortions in the third trimester are done in one of two ways: extraction or induction. If extraction is used, the cervix is dilated with laminaria, and the fetus is extracted with forceps and other surgical instruments. With induction, laminaria are also used, but women are given drugs that cause the uterus to contract, and the fetus is then expelled or "delivered." Both procedures have been shown to be safe and humane. The risk of complications is about the same as for giving birth.

Note: Intact dilation and extraction is a variation of the basic extraction procedure and is used for both second- and third-trimester abortions. After dilation, the fetus is turned and partially extracted in a breech, feet-first, position. Fluid is then drained from the head and the skull compressed to complete the extraction. Doctors who use the procedure say it reduces the likelihood of damage to the cervix so that women can carry future pregnancies to term. At present, it is estimated that IDEs account for less than 1 percent of all abortions done in the United States each year.

Third-Trimester Abortions

Third-trimester, or late, abortions are usually 2-to-3-day procedures. Costs range from around $1,700 to over $7,000. Depending on how long you have been pregnant, you will need two to five appointments for laminaria insertion. The abortion will be performed on the second or third day, once the cervix is dilated wide enough to ensure that the fetus can be safely extracted or expelled.

Insertion of the laminaria is sometimes done with IV sedation—an increased number of laminaria will be inserted each time—and cramping and other physical discomfort may occur between appointments. In most cases, you will be given pain medication for cramps, and you will need to stay near the clinic and have direct access to a telephone to ensure that emergency treatment can be arranged immediately if any complications develop. Most providers have special arrangements with local hotels. Information on reservations and your appointments at the clinic will be kept strictly confidential.

In most cases, fetal demise occurs the first day of laminaria insertion. The drugs most commonly used are digoxin and lidocaine, and they are injected directly into the uterus.

Once dilation is complete, late abortions usually take 2 to 4 hours and are performed with IV sedation or a general anesthetic. Recovery time at the clinic may be 2 hours or longer. You will receive detailed instructions on aftercare, including how to monitor yourself for signs of infection or other complications and what to do if your breasts start producing milk, which may occur a few days after the abortion.

Seeing the Fetus or Fetal Remains

For some couples, seeing the fetus or fetal remains after an abortion can be an important part of accepting the loss of a pregnancy and beginning to grieve. While asking to see or hold the fetus is no longer considered an abnormal request, policies and specific arrangements will vary from provider to provider. In some cases, your doctor or a counselor at the clinic will talk with you directly about viewing the fetus after the abortion; in other cases, the subject will not be brought up unless you ask about it.

Whether you see the body or remains—tissue and body parts—of the fetus will depend on how long you have been pregnant and the procedure your provider uses. Women who are less than 24 to 25 weeks pregnant and have a regular D & E will view fetal remains. In such cases, additional counseling may be recommended, or you may be required to look at a book with written descriptions and pictures of fetal remains so you will be prepared physically and emotionally for what you're going to see.

If you are having a third-trimester abortion—extraction or induction—in most cases you will be able to see the body of the fetus. Clinics that perform third-trimester abortions often talk with couples about whether they wish to see the fetus, or "baby," after the abortion and what arrangements they wish to make for cremation or burial of the body. Private rooms are usually available for couples who want to see and hold the baby, and you can bring baby clothes, toys, and a camera. In most instances, clinic staff will bathe and dress the baby so physical defects are not visible. You can also ask other family members to be present for support or grieving.

Note: After a third-trimester abortion, some couples may wish to have a funeral or other memorial event for the baby, or the provider may arrange for cremation or other humane disposal of the body. Arrangements will vary from provider to provider. You should ask your doctor or clinic about their policies.

GRIEVING AND GETTING SUPPORT

For many couples, interrupting a wanted pregnancy represents a painful and seemingly irreplaceable loss, and like any parents mourning for a much-loved child, you and your partner may need to grieve and talk about what has happened. Unfortunately, the emotional needs of couples are often overlooked or misunderstood at this time, and many end up feeling isolated and without support. You may be told you should "recover" or "put the experience behind you" in a few weeks or months. Even well-meaning friends and family members may seem insensitive or uncomfortable at any mention of the abortion or similar topics, such as pregnancy or a relative's new baby.

What most women and their partners find is that grieving is an ongoing and intensely personal process. Your emotional needs at this time will depend on a range of factors, such as religious or spiritual beliefs about life and death and how you express your feelings—individually and as a couple. For some women and their partners, naming the baby or seeing it after the abortion may seem too painful or gruesome, while for others, taking pictures of the baby or even having a funeral or some other memorial event may help ease feelings of loss and grief.

Getting support is essential—especially after the initial shock and trauma of the lost pregnancy is over. You can expect feelings of sadness, emptiness, depression, and anger to resurface at key times throughout the first year, such as your original due date or the first Thanksgiving or major holiday after the abortion, and you may want to spend these days alone or with a few close friends or family members. Some couples also plan personal rituals or memorial ceremonies for the anniversary of the abortion itself, which they commemorate as the lost child's birthday.

In recent years, women who have had late abortions have begun to reach out to each other, and support groups for women and couples are now available. To find a group in your area, ask your doctor, clergy, clinic, or a local hospital. Another good source of information is *A Heartbreaking Choice,* a monthly newsletter with listings of national organizations, local support groups, and on-line resources for couples who have terminated a wanted pregnancy. You can contact them at Pineapple Press, P.O. Box 312, St. Johns, MI 48879; 616-627-4296.

"IT GAVE US TIME TO SAY GOOD-BYE": SARAH'S STORY

▼   Sarah's story illustrates how a fetal anomaly can go undiscovered until late in a pregnancy and why, for some families, late abortion can be a loving and humane choice. Sarah was in the 8th month of her third pregnancy when her doctor noticed she was losing weight and recommended an ultrasound, "just to be safe." The results, she recalls, were devastating.

> I had the ultrasound, and the doctor said there was something terribly wrong. What he found is called an encephalocele, which can range in severity, but in my case, it meant two-thirds of my daughter's brain had grown outside her skull. When I felt her kicking, she was actually having convulsions and seizures because of the compression on the part of her brain that was outside of her body, and she was in critical and dangerous physical condition.

Although Sarah and her husband, Jack, were both health care professionals, at first neither were aware that they might be able to terminate the pregnancy. After consulting with a geneticist, however, they were referred to a clinic that specializes in late abortions.

> My husband and I were adamant that we would not let her be born if it meant she was going to suffer—like she would be born and then be gasping for air, and they would have to put her on life support systems. We couldn't subject ourselves, or the baby, to the unknown, so the abortion was the choice that gave us the most control.

Sarah and Jack spoke with the doctor and a counselor at the clinic before leaving home. They were told they and their two children—then 8 and 10—could see the baby after the abortion, and they were encouraged to bring baby clothes and a camera. The procedure itself, Sarah says, took 3 days.

> The clinic was this beautiful, havenlike place. We went there twice a day for the laminaria, and they knocked me out with an IV sedation, which was great because I couldn't sleep otherwise. Afterward we would go back to the hotel, and I would feel cramping, like mild menstrual cramps. The time before the actual abortion was so important because it gave us time to say good-bye to her. It was the worst time in my life; my husband would hold my belly during those last nights.

Sarah believes her daughter—whom she and Jack named Andrea—died the day before the procedure. The doctor was concerned that the abortion might cause damage to Sarah's cervix, and an IDE was performed.

The fine line between when she did or didn't die, I really don't care about. I know whenever she did die, she didn't feel it. I went back to the clinic and was knocked out, and when I woke up, she was there, and so was the rest of my family. It was devastating when they first brought her in. I was almost afraid to look at her, and I was afraid to hold her because I knew I wouldn't want to let her go. We ended up passing her around, letting everyone be with her. My son had made her a bracelet and brought a stuffed animal to give her, and the kids held her a few times. As difficult and painful as it was, it was the best thing. We took pictures and we grieved as a family, and I cherish those pictures now. We also had a funeral, and almost two hundred people showed up.

Following the abortion, Sarah says she was "obsessed" with memories of Andrea for several months and suffered periods of deep depression. She and Jack also talked with a counselor during this time and received support from friends and family members.

I built a little shrine to her with all her baby clothes and gifts. I would go to the grocery store and not buy anything, just walk up and down the aisles, looking and knowing I was supposed to buy something, and cry and cry. What got me through were my kids, because I had to stay sane for them. The day-to-day activities with them—driving them to music lessons and soccer—saved my life. Our friends took care of us too, taking the kids at a minute's notice when I was sick and Jack was working. The fact that I wasn't alone is what got me through.

Since her abortion, Sarah has spoken publicly about her experience. She is one of several women who testified before Congress in 1996, during hearings on a law to ban the IDE procedure. The bill passed Congress but was vetoed by President Clinton. Since then, several states have enacted laws banning IDE. Some of these laws have been overturned or ruled unconstitutional; some are currently in force, and a federal ban is again being considered.

LATE ABORTION:
AT A GLANCE

• Abortion after the 24th or 25th week of pregnancy is illegal in most states, except in cases where a fetal anomaly has been diagnosed or continuing the pregnancy would put a woman's life at risk. About 600 late abortions are performed in the United States each year.

- Fetal anomalies, or defects, occur in 1 to 2 percent of all pregnancies. In many cases they are *not* caused by genetic factors or anything a couple did before or during a pregnancy. Most defects cannot be diagnosed until the second or third trimester.

- If an anomaly is found, you will receive counseling on the severity of the defect and whether the fetus will survive if born alive. If you decide to terminate the pregnancy, you will be referred to a late-abortion provider. You can also call the NAF referral line at 800-772-9100.

- Clinics that perform late abortions often provide special services, such as private waiting rooms for women and their partners. If you need something, *ask for it.*

- For abortions before the 24th or 25th weeks of pregnancy, a regular dilation and evacuation (D & E) will be performed. Laminaria are used to dilate the cervix slowly over a 1-to-2-day period, and the fetus is removed with vacuum aspiration, forceps, and curettage.

- The term "partial birth" abortion and antichoice claims that some late abortion procedures are inhumane are medically incorrect. In many cases, drugs are used to stop fetal heartbeat, and *the fetus is not alive at the time of procedure.*

- Two methods are used for third-trimester abortions—extraction or induction. With extraction, the cervix is dilated with laminaria, and the fetus is removed with forceps and other surgical instruments. Laminaria are also used for induction, but the woman is given drugs that cause the uterus to contract, and the fetus is expelled, or "delivered."

- Intact dilation and extraction—what antichoicers call "partial birth" abortion—accounts for less than 1 percent of all U.S. abortions. During the procedure, the fetus is extracted feet first, and its skull is partially drained and compressed, which, some doctors say, prevents damage to the cervix.

- Clinics that perform late abortions may also arrange for cremation or other humane disposal of the fetus. After the abortion, you and your partner can also see the fetus or fetal remains.

- For many couples, having a late abortion is similar to losing a child. *Get support and allow yourself to grieve.* Information on support groups is available from *A Heartbreaking Choice,* a monthly newsletter for couples who have interrupted a wanted pregnancy.

This appendix provides a brief summary of current state abortion laws and the phone number of one prochoice organization women can call for information and referrals on abortion and counseling services in their state. The information on state laws is based on the 1997 edition of *Who Decides: A State-by-State Review of Abortion and Reproductive Rights,* published by the NARAL Foundation. A "No" indicates that the state has no law of this type on the books or it is currently not being enforced. Unless otherwise noted, all parental notification and consent laws apply to minors under 18. State laws are subject to change. For up-to-date information on the laws in your state, contact your clinic or a NARAL affiliate.

Alabama

* *Informed consent/waiting period:* No
* *Parental notification/consent:* One-parent consent or judicial bypass.
* *Public funding:* Life endangerment only
* *Clinic access:* No
* *Information and referrals:* **Planned Parenthood of Alabama, 205-322-2121**

Alaska

* *Informed consent/waiting period:* No
* *Parental notification/consent:* No
* *Public funding:* All or most circumstances
* *Clinic access:* No
* *Information and referrals:* **Planned Parenthood of Alaska, 907-277-4822**

Arizona

* *Informed consent/waiting period:* No
* *Parental notification/consent:* No
* *Public funding:* Life endangerment, rape, and incest only

* *Clinic access:* No
* *Information and referrals:* **Planned Parenthood of Central and Northern Arizona, 602-277-7526**

Arkansas

* *Informed consent/waiting period:* No
* *Parental notification/consent:* Two-parent notification with 48-hour waiting period or judicial bypass
* *Public funding:* Life endangerment, rape, and incest only
* *Clinic access:* No
* *Information and referrals:* **Planned Parenthood of Greater Arkansas, 501-666-7526**

California

* *Informed consent/waiting period:* No
* *Parental notification/consent:* No
* *Public funding:* All or most circumstances
* *Clinic access:* Obstructing or blocking access to a clinic is a misdemeanor; arson, vandalism, and butyric acid attacks are felonies; individuals who are harassed can sue for damages
* *Information and referrals:* **Access, 800-376-4636**

Colorado

* *Informed consent/waiting period:* No
* *Parental notification/consent:* No
* *Public funding:* Life endangerment, rape, and incest only
* *Clinic access:* Picketers must stay 8 feet away from anyone within a 100-foot safety zone surrounding clinics; violation of law is a misdemeanor; individuals who are harassed can sue for damages
* *Information and referrals:* **Religious Coalition for Reproductive Choice, 303-756-9996**

Connecticut

* *Informed consent/waiting period:* No
* *Parental notification/consent:* Counseling on reproductive options and the possibility of adult involvement required for all minors under 16
* *Public funding:* All or most circumstances
* *Clinic access:* No
* *Information and referrals:* **INFOLINE, 800-203-1234**

Delaware

* *Informed consent/waiting period:* No
* *Parental notification/consent:* Under 16, one-parent notification with 24-hour waiting period or judicial bypass; notification not required if teen receives counseling from grandparent or licensed mental health professional not employed by clinic

+ *Public funding:* Life endangerment, rape, and incest only
+ *Clinic access:* No
+ *Information and referrals:* **Planned Parenthood of Delaware, 302-655-7296**

District of Columbia

+ *Informed consent/waiting period:* No
+ *Parental notification/consent:* No
+ *Public funding:* All or most circumstances
+ *Clinic access:* Any attempt to obstruct or prevent access to a clinic is a misdemeanor
+ *Information and referrals:* **Planned Parenthood of Metropolitan Washington, 202-347-8512**

Florida

+ *Informed consent/waiting period:* No
+ *Parental notification/consent:* No
+ *Public funding:* Life endangerment, rape, and incest only
+ *Clinic access:* No
+ *Information and referrals:* **Florida Abortion Council, 800-432-8517**

Georgia

+ *Informed consent/waiting period:* No
+ *Parental notification/consent:* One-parent notification with 24-hour waiting period or judicial bypass
+ *Public funding:* Life endangerment, rape, and incest only
+ *Clinic access:* No
+ *Information and referrals:* **Planned Parenthood of Georgia, 404-688-9300**

Hawaii

+ *Informed consent/waiting period:* No
+ *Parental notification/consent:* No
+ *Public funding:* All or most circumstances
+ *Clinic access:* No
+ *Information and referrals:* **Planned Parenthood of Hawaii, 808-235-8997**

Idaho

+ *Informed consent/waiting period:* "If reasonably possible," women must receive state-prepared materials including photographs and descriptions of fetal development at 2-week intervals, a list of public and private agencies providing assistance for pregnant women and children, descriptions of abortion procedures, and the risks of abortion and childbirth; 24-hour waiting period
+ *Parental notification/consent:* One-parent notification with 24-hour waiting period "if reasonably possible"; no judicial bypass
+ *Public funding:* All or most circumstances with certification by two physicians that the abortion is necessary to preserve a woman's life or health
+ *Clinic access:* No
+ *Information and referrals:* **Planned Parenthood of Idaho, 208-376-9300**

Illinois

• *Informed consent/waiting period:* No
• *Parental notification/consent:* No
• *Public funding:* All or most circumstances
• *Clinic access:* No
• *Information and referrals:* **Planned Parenthood Association, 312-427-2275**

Indiana

• *Informed consent/waiting period:* No
• *Parental notification/consent:* One-parent consent or judicial bypass
• *Public funding:* Life endangerment, rape, and incest
• *Clinic access:* No
• *Information and referrals:* **Women's Pavilion, 219-272-1010**

Iowa

• *Informed consent/waiting period:* No
• *Parental notification/consent:* No
• *Public funding:* Life endangerment, rape, incest, and in some cases, fetal deformity
• *Clinic access:* No
• *Information and referrals:* **Planned Parenthood of Greater Iowa, 800-568-2404**

Kansas

• *Informed consent/waiting period:* State-mandated materials include a description of the abortion procedure, alternatives to abortion, the risks of abortion and childbirth, the gestational age of the fetus, and community resources available for pregnant women; 24-hour waiting period
• *Parental notification/consent:* One-parent notification or judicial bypass, and mandatory reproductive options counseling
• *Public funding:* Life endangerment, rape, and incest
• *Clinic harassment:* Interference with access to a clinic is criminal trespass
• *Information and referrals:* **Planned Parenthood of Kansas, 316-263-7575**

Kentucky

• *Informed consent/waiting period:* No
• *Parental notification/consent:* One-parent consent or judicial bypass
• *Public funding:* Life endangerment, rape, and incest
• *Clinic access:* No
• *Information and referrals:* **Religious Coalition for Reproductive Choice, 502-222-7940**

Louisiana

• *Informed consent/waiting period:* State-mandated lecture and booklets contain information on abortion procedure, alternatives to abortion, the gestational age of fetus, risks of abortion and childbirth, the name of doctor who will perform the abortion, and community resources available to pregnant women; 24-hour waiting period and face-to-face session with doctor required

* *Parental notification/consent:* One-parent consent or judicial bypass
* *Public funding:* Life endangerment, rape, and incest
* *Clinic access:* No
* *Information and referrals:* **Planned Parenthood of Louisiana, 504-891-8013**

Maine

* *Informed consent/waiting period:* No
* *Parental notification/consent:* Consent of one parent or adult family member, judicial bypass, or reproductive options counseling from a physician, nurse, physician's assistant, or qualified counselor.
* *Public funding:* Life endangerment, rape, and incest
* *Clinic access:* Physical obstruction of clinic buildings, vandalism, or interference with clinic services is a misdemeanor
* *Information and referrals:* **Planned Parenthood of Northern New England, 207-874-1095**

Maryland

* *Informed consent/waiting period:* No
* *Parental notification/consent:* One-parent notification or physician bypass
* *Public funding:* All or most circumstances
* *Clinic access:* Obstructing, impeding, or hindering access to a clinic is a misdemeanor
* *Information and referrals:* **Planned Parenthood Association of Maryland, 410-576-1400**

Massachusetts

* *Informed consent/waiting period:* No
* *Parental notification/consent:* Two-parent consent or judicial bypass
* *Public funding:* All of most circumstances
* *Clinic access:* Obstructing access to a clinic or impeding provision of services is a misdemeanor
* *Information and referrals:* **Planned Parenthood League of Massachusetts, 800-682-9218** (in Massachusetts only) **or 617-731-2525**

Michigan

* *Informed consent/waiting period:* No
* *Parental notification/consent:* One-parent consent or judicial bypass
* *Public funding:* Life endangerment, rape, or incest
* *Clinic access:* No
* *Information and referrals:* **Planned Parenthood Affiliates of Michigan, 517-482-1080**

Minnesota

+ *Informed consent/waiting period:* No
+ *Parental notification/consent:* Two-parent notification with 48-hour waiting period or judicial bypass.
+ *Public funding:* All or most circumstances
+ *Clinic access:* Obstructing access to a clinic is a misdemeanor; individuals who are harassed may sue for damages
+ *Information and referrals:* **Planned Parenthood of Minnesota, 612-698-2406**

Mississippi

+ *Informed consent/waiting period:* State-mandated lecture and booklets contain information on fetal development and probable gestational age of fetus, risks of abortion and carrying pregnancy to term, availability of community resources for pregnant women; 24-hour waiting period and face-to-face session with doctor required
+ *Parental notification/consent:* Two-parent consent or judicial bypass
+ *Public funding:* Life endangerment only
+ *Clinic access:* No
+ *Information and referrals:* **Jackson Women's Health Organization, 601-366-2261**

Missouri

+ *Informed consent/waiting period:* No
+ *Parental notification/consent:* One-parent consent or judicial bypass
+ *Public funding:* Life endangerment, rape, or incest
+ *Clinic access:* No
+ *Information and referrals:* **Missouri Religious Coalition for Reproductive Choice, 800-204-0691 or 314-721-2446**

Montana

+ *Informed consent/waiting period:* No
+ *Parental notification/consent:* One-parent notification with 48-hour waiting period or judicial bypass
+ *Public funding:* All or most circumstances
+ *Clinic access:* No
+ *Information and referrals:* **Intermountain Planned Parenthood, 406-248-3636**

Nebraska

+ *Informed consent/waiting period:* State-mandated lecture and booklets contain information on fetal development and probable gestational age of fetus, risks of abortion and carrying pregnancy to term, the name of the physician who will perform the abortion, and the availability of community resources for pregnant women; 24-hour waiting period
+ *Parental notification/consent:* One-parent notification with 48-hour waiting period or judicial bypass
+ *Public funding:* Life endangerment, rape, or incest

* *Clinic access:* No
* *Information and referrals:* **Planned Parenthood of Omaha, 402-554-1045**

Nevada

* *Informed consent/waiting period:* No
* *Parental notification/consent:* No
* *Public funding:* Life endangerment, rape, or incest
* *Clinic access:* Preventing or obstructing access to a clinic is a misdemeanor
* *Information and referrals:* **Planned Parenthood of Northern Nevada, 702-688-5555**

New Hampshire

* *Informed consent/waiting period:* No
* *Parental notification/consent:* No
* *Public funding:* Life endangerment, rape, or incest
* *Clinic access:* No
* *Information and referrals:* **Feminist Health Center, 603-225-2739**

New Jersey

* *Informed consent/waiting period:* No
* *Parental notification/consent:* No
* *Public funding:* All or most circumstances
* *Clinic access:* No
* *Information and referrals:* **Religious Coalition for Reproductive Choice, 201-895-8883**

New Mexico

* *Informed consent/waiting period:* No
* *Parental notification/consent:* No
* *Public funding:* All or most circumstances
* *Clinic access:* No
* *Information and referrals:* **NARAL New Mexico/Right to Choose, 505-878-9576**

New York

* *Informed consent/waiting period:* No
* *Parental notification/consent:* No
* *Public funding:* All or most circumstances
* *Clinic access:* No
* *Information and referrals:* **New York State NARAL, 212-343-0114**; e-mail: naralny@aol.com

North Carolina

* *Informed consent/waiting period:* No
* *Parental notification/consent:* Consent of one parent or a grandparent with whom the teen has been living for at least 6 months or judicial bypass

- *Public funding:* Life endangerment, rape, or incest
- *Clinic access:* Obstruction of health care facilities, threat or injury to patients or health care providers, and possessing a dangerous weapon at a demonstration at a clinic are misdemeanors; individuals who are harassed or injured may sue for damages
- *Information and referrals:* **Planned Parenthood of Orange and Durham Counties, 919-942-7762**

North Dakota

- *Informed consent/waiting period:* State-mandated lecture and booklets contain information on fetal development and probable gestational age of fetus, the risks of abortion and carrying the pregnancy to term, the name of the physician who will perform the abortion, and the availability of community resources for pregnant women; 24-hour waiting period
- *Parental notification/consent:* Two-parent consent or judicial bypass
- *Public funding:* Life endangerment, rape, or incest
- *Clinic access:* No
- *Information and referrals:* **Fargo Women's Health Center, 701-235-0999**

Ohio

- *Informed consent/waiting period:* State-mandated lecture and booklets contain information on fetal development and probable gestational age of the fetus, the risks of abortion and carrying the pregnancy to term, the name of the physician who will perform the abortion, and the availability of community resources for pregnant women; 24-hour waiting period
- *Parental notification/consent:* Notification of one parent or, in some circumstances, a grandparent, stepparent or brother or sister over 21, with 24-hour waiting period or judicial bypass
- *Public funding:* Life endangerment, rape, or incest
- *Clinic access:* No
- *Information and referrals:* **NARAL of Ohio, 800-466-2725**

Oklahoma

- *Informed consent/waiting period:* No
- *Parental notification/consent:* No
- *Public funding:* Life endangerment, rape, or incest
- *Clinic access:* No
- *Information and referrals:* **Planned Parenthood of Eastern Oklahoma, 918-587-1101**

Oregon

- *Informed consent/waiting period:* No
- *Parental notification/consent:* No
- *Public funding:* All or most circumstances
- *Clinic access:* Damage to a medical facility or interference with medical services is a felony
- *Information and referrals:* **Oregon NARAL Abortion Provider Helpline, 503-294-9097**

Pennsylvania

♦ *Informed consent/waiting period:* State-mandated lectures and booklets contain information on fetal development and the probable gestational age of the fetus, the risks of abortion and carrying the pregnancy to term, and the availability of community resources for pregnant women; 24-hour waiting period and face-to-face meeting with doctor required
♦ *Parental notification/consent:* One-parent consent or judicial bypass
♦ *Public funding:* Life endangerment, rape, or incest
♦ *Clinic access:* No
♦ *Information and referrals:* **Choice, 800-848-3367 (in Pennsylvania only) or 215-985-3355**

Rhode Island

♦ *Informed consent/waiting period:* No
♦ *Parental notification/consent:* One-parent consent or judicial bypass
♦ *Public funding:* Life endangerment, rape, or incest
♦ *Clinic access:* No
♦ *Information and referrals:* **Planned Parenthood of Rhode Island, 401-421-9620**

South Carolina

♦ *Informed consent/waiting period:* State-mandated materials contain information on fetal development and the probable gestational age of the fetus, the risks of abortion and carrying the pregnancy to term, and the availability of community resources for pregnant women; 1-hour waiting period
♦ *Parental notification/consent:* For unemancipated minors under 17, consent of one parent or grandparent or judicial bypass
♦ *Public funding:* Life endangerment, rape, or incest
♦ *Clinic access:* No
♦ *Information and referrals:* **Planned Parenthood of Central South Carolina, 803-256-4908**

South Dakota

♦ *Informed consent/waiting period:* State-mandated lecture and booklets contain information on fetal development and the probable gestational age of the fetus, the risks of abortion and carrying the pregnancy to term, and the availability of community resources for pregnant women; 24-hour waiting period
♦ *Parental notification/consent:* One-parent notification or judicial bypass
♦ *Public funding:* Life endangerment only
♦ *Clinic access:* No
♦ *Information and referrals:* **Planned Parenthood of South Dakota, 800-314-7216 or 605-361-5100**

Tennessee

♦ *Informed consent/waiting period:* No
♦ *Parental notification/consent:* No
♦ *Public funding:* Life endangerment, rape, or incest

+ *Clinic access:* No
+ *Information and referrals:* **Planned Parenthood of Nashville, 615-321-7216**

Texas

+ *Informed consent/waiting period:* No
+ *Parental notification/consent:* No
+ *Public funding:* Life endangerment, rape, or incest
+ *Clinic access:* No
+ *Information and referrals:* **Texas Family Planning Association, 512-448-4857**

Utah

+ *Informed consent/waiting period:* State-mandated lecture, booklets, and video contain information on fetal development and the probable gestational age of the fetus, the risks of abortion and carrying the pregnancy to term, and the availability of community resources for pregnant women; 24-hour waiting period and face-to-face session with doctor, nurse, nurse-midwife, or physician's assistant required
+ *Parental notification/consent:* Two-parent notification; no judicial bypass
+ *Public funding:* Life endangerment, rape, or incest
+ *Clinic access:* No
+ *Information and referrals:* **Utah Women's Clinic, 801-531-9192**

Vermont

+ *Informed consent/waiting period:* No
+ *Parental notification/consent:* No
+ *Public funding:* All or most circumstances
+ *Clinic access:* No
+ *Information and referrals:* **Vermont Women's Health Center, 802-863-1386**

Virginia

+ *Informed consent/waiting period:* No
+ *Parental notification/consent:* One-parent notification with 24-hour waiting period or judicial bypass; physician bypass allowed in cases of sexual abuse
+ *Public funding:* Life endangerment, rape, or incest
+ *Clinic access:* No
+ *Information and referrals:* **Virginia League of Planned Parenthood, 804-788-6742**

Washington

+ *Informed consent/waiting period:* No
+ *Parental notification/consent:* No
+ *Public funding:* All or most circumstances
+ *Clinic access:* Obstruction of medical facilities and threats or injury to patients or staff are misdemeanors
+ *Information and referrals:* **Planned Parenthood of Seattle-King County, 800-324-7087 (in Washington only) or 206-328-7734**

West Virginia

- *Informed consent/waiting period:* No
- *Parental notification/consent:* One-parent notification with 24-hour waiting period, or physician or judicial bypass
- *Public funding:* All or most circumstances
- *Clinic access:* No
- *Information and referrals:* **Planned Parenthood of West Virginia, 304-295-3331**

Wisconsin

- *Informed consent/waiting period:* No
- *Parental notification/consent:* Consent of one parent or a grandparent, aunt, uncle, or sibling over the age of 25 or judicial bypass
- *Public funding:* Life endangerment, rape, or incest
- *Clinic access:* Entering a medical facility "under circumstances tending to provoke a breach of the peace" is a misdemeanor
- *Information and referrals:* **Planned Parenthood of Wisconsin, 800-472-2703 (in Wisconsin only)**

Wyoming

- *Informed consent/waiting period:* No
- *Parental notification/consent:* One-parent consent with 48-hour waiting period or judicial bypass
- *Public funding:* Life endangerment, rape, or incest
- *Clinic access:* No
- *Information and referrals:* **Planned Parenthood of the Rocky Mountains, 307-234-1669**

APPENDIX 2

RESOURCES

AND

BIBLIOGRAPHY

Resources

Abortion Access Project
552 Massachusetts Avenue, Ste. 215
Cambridge, MA 02139
617-494-1161
Organization working to increase the number of hospitals providing abortion services.

Abortion Clinics OnLine
e-mail: feedback@gynpages.com
Web site: http://www.gynpages.com
Referrals to selected clinics, information on abortion and women's health, and links to other prochoice and women's organizations and publications.

Abortion Rights Activist Home Page
e-mail: agm@cais.com
Web site: http://www.cais.com/agm/main/index.htlm
Good starting place to find out about abortion and reproductive health issues on the World Wide Web; up-to-date news on abortion issues and links to other organizations.

Alan Guttmacher Institute
111 Fifth Avenue
New York, NY 10003
212-248-1111
e-mail: info@agi-usa.org
Web site: http://www.agi-usa.org/
Research and publications on abortion and reproductive health issues.

American Civil Liberties Union Reproductive Freedom Project
132 West 43rd Street
New York, NY 10036
212-944-9800, ext. 618
e-mail: rfpaclu@aol.com

Web site: http://www.aclu.org
Information and legal action on abortion and other reproductive health issues; local chapters can provide referrals to prochoice lawyers.

Body Politic
P.O. Box 2363
Binghamton, NY 13902-2363
607-648-2760
e-mail: annebower@delphi.com
Web site: http://www.bodypolitic.org/default.htm
Monthly journal on abortion politics in the United States; Web site features national directory of prochoice organizations.

Bridging the Gap Communications, Inc.
P.O. Box 33218
Decatur, GA 30033
800-721-6990
Information and publications on emergency contraception, birth control, and sex education.

Center for Reproductive Law and Policy
120 Wall Street, 18th Floor
New York, NY 10005
212-514-5534
e-mail: crlp@echonyc.com
Clearinghouse for information on federal and state laws and policy on abortion and reproductive health issues.

Emergency Contraception Hotline
800-584-9911
Web site: http://opr.princeton.edu/ec/
Information on emergency contraception and referrals to clinics and other providers.

Feminist Majority Foundation
1600 Wilson Boulevard
Arlington, VA 22219
703-522-2214
e-mail: femmaj@aol.com
Web site: http://www.feminist.org/home.html
Information and political action on abortion, clinic violence, and other political issues affecting women; Web site features Feminist Internet Gateway with links to hundreds of women's groups and resources.

National Abortion and Reproductive Rights Action League
1156 15th Street, NW
Washington, DC 20005
202-973-3000
e-mail: naral@newmedium.com
Web site: http://www.naral.org
Information and political action on abortion and reproductive health care issues.

National Abortion Federation
1755 Massachusetts Avenue, NW
Suite 600
Washington, DC 20036
202-667-5881
800-772-9100 (U.S.)
800-424-2280 (Canada)
e-mail: naf@prochoice.org
Web site: http://www.prochoice.org/naf
National organization of abortion providers; information on abortion, clinics, and state laws; national referral line.

National Network of Abortion Funds
c/o CLPP
Hampshire College
Hampshire, MA 01002
413-582-5645
e-mail: clpp@hamp.hampshire.edu (Put NNAF on subject line.)
Web site: http://hamp.hampshire.edu/~clpp/nnaf
National organization of abortion assistance funds.

Pineapple Press
P.O. Box 312
St. Johns, MI 48879
517-224-1881
Publications for women and couples who have interrupted a wanted pregnancy.

Planned Parenthood Federation of America
810 Seventh Avenue
New York, NY 10019
212-541-7800
800-230-7526
e-mail: communications@ppfa.org
Web site: http://www.ppfa.org/ppfa/
National organization of nonprofit reproductive health care clinics offering information, counseling, and comprehensive reproductive health care; national clinic referral line.

Population Council
One Dag Hammarskjold Plaza
New York, NY 10017
212-339-0500
e-mail: pubinfo@popcouncil.org
Web site: http://www.popcouncil.org
Research and information on medical abortion and mifepristone (RU-486).

Prochoice Resources
3255 Hennepin Avenue
Suite 255
Minneapolis, MN 55408
612-825-2000

e-mail: choicemn@aol.com
Educational materials on abortion and reproductive health care issues.

Rape, Abuse and Incest National Network
800-656-4673
National referral line that automatically switches callers to a local rape crisis center; information on confidentiality and sexual abuse reporting laws.

Religious Coalition for Reproductive Choice
1025 Vermont Avenue, NW
Suite 1130
Washington, DC 20005
202-628-7700
e-mail: info@rcrc.org
Web site: www.rcrc.org
National organization of prochoice clergy, churches, and synagogues; local chapters can provide referrals for spiritual counseling.

Bibliography

Alan Guttmacher Institute. "Facts in Brief: Abortion in the United States." New York, 1995.

———. "Issues in Brief: Lawmakers Grapple With Parents' Role in Teen Access to Reproductive Health Care." New York, 1995.

American Civil Liberties Union Reproductive Freedom Project. *Parental Notice Laws: Their Catastrophic Impact on Teenagers' Right to Abortion.* New York, 1986.

Baker, Anne. *How to Cope Successfully after an Abortion.* Hope Clinic for Women, Granite City, Ill., 1992.

———. *How to Cope With Guilt.* Hope Clinic for Women, Granite City, Ill., 1982.

———. *"I'll Never Have Sex Again!"* Hope Clinic for Women, Granite City, Ill., 1995.

Bonavoglia, Angela, ed. *The Choices We Made: Twenty-five Women and Men Speak Out about Abortion.* Random House, New York, 1991.

Boston Women's Health Book Collective. *The New Our Bodies, Ourselves.* Simon & Schuster, New York, 1992.

Centers for Disease Control. "Abortion Surveillance: Preliminary Data, United States, 1994." *Morbidity and Mortality Weekly Report.* January 3, 1997.

Chalker, Rebecca, and Carol Downer. *A Woman's Book of Choices: Abortion, Menstrual Extraction, RU-486.* Four Walls Eight Windows, New York, 1992.

Cooper, Marc. "Robbing the Cradle: The Christian Right's Adoption Racket." *Village Voice.* July 26, 1994.

de Jung, Trilby, Scott Caplan-Cotenoff, Susan Holman, Amy Fairchild Carrino, and Dennis de Leon. "HIV-Related Discrimination in Abortion Clinics, New York City, USA, 1988–1992." Poster and paper presented at the International AIDS Conference, Berlin, June 1993.

Derenge, Sara, and Nancy L. James. *A Guide to Fetal Development for Abortion Providers.* Center for Choice II, Toledo, Ohio, 1993.

———. *A Guide to Fetal Development for Abortion Providers: The Second Trimester (14 to 20 weeks LMP).* Center for Choice II, Toledo, Ohio, 1993.

Donovan, Patricia. *Our Daughters' Decisions: The Conflict in State Law on Abortion and Other Issues.* Alan Guttmacher Institute, New York, 1992.

———. *The Politics of Blame: Family Planning, Abortion and the Poor.* Alan Guttmacher Institute, New York, 1995.

Eggebroten, Anne. *Abortion, My Choice, God's Grace: Christian Women Tell Their Stories.* New Paradigm Books, Pasadena, Calif., 1994.

Eisenberg, Arlene, Heidi E. Murkoff, and Sandee E. Hathaway. *What to Expect When You're Expecting.* Workman Publishing, New York, 1991.

Feminist Majority Foundation. *1995 Clinic Violence Survey Report.* Arlington, Va., 1996.

———. *1996 Clinic Violence Survey Report.* Arlington, Va., 1997.

Ferreyra, Susan, and Katrine Hughes. *Table Manners: A Guide to the Pelvic Examination for Disabled Women and Health Care Providers.* Planned Parenthood Golden Gate, San Francisco, 1982.

Fried, Marlene Gerber. *From Abortion to Reproductive Freedom: Transforming a Movement.* South End Press, Boston, 1990.

Gardner, Joy. *A Difficult Decision: A Compassionate Book about Abortion,* 2d ed. Crossing Press, Freedom, Calif., 1986.

Goodroe, Morgan. *Abortion Resolution Workbook: Ways to Connect Head and Heart.* Routh Street Women's Clinic, Dallas, Tex.

Hatcher, Robert A., James Trussell, Felicia Stewart, Susan Howells, Caroline Russell, and Deborah Kowel. *Emergency Contraception: The Nation's Best Kept Secret.* Bridging the Gap Communications, Decatur, Ga., 1995.

Henshaw, Stanley K., and Jennifer Van Vort, eds. *The Abortion Factbook, 1992 Edition: Readings, Trends, and State and Local Data to 1988.* Alan Guttmacher Institute, New York, 1992.

Hern, Warren M. *Abortion Practice.* J.B. Lippincott Company, Philadelphia, Pa., 1984.

Hope Medical Group for Women. *After Your Abortion . . . A Natural Response.* Granite City, Ill.

Hoshiko, Sumi. *Our Choices: Women's Personal Decisions about Abortion.* Harrington Park Press, Binghamton, N.Y., 1993.

Lyon, Wendy L., with Molly A. Minnick. *A Mother's Dilemma.* Pineapple Press, St. Johns, Mich., 1993.

Minnick, Molly A., Kathleen J. Delp, and Mary C. Ciotti. *A Time to Decide, A Time to Heal: For Parents Making Difficult Decisions about Babies They Love,* 4th ed. Pineapple Press, St. Johns, Mich., 1994.

Mississippi Department of Health. *Informed Consent Information and Resources.* Jackson, Miss., 1995.

National Abortion and Reproductive Rights Action League Foundation. *Who Decides: A State-by-State Review of Abortion and Reproductive Rights,* 6th ed. Washington, D.C., 1997.

National Abortion Federation. "How and When: A Medical Abortion Update." Washington, D.C., 1996.

———. *Parental Involvement Laws: A Guide For Providers.* Washington, D.C., 1991.

———. *Standards for Abortion Care.* Washington, D.C., 1988.

———. *The Truth about Abortion: A Fact Sheet Series.* Washington, D.C., 1991.

———. *Undue Burdens: The States' Experiences.* Washington, D.C., 1993.

National Network of Abortion Funds. *Legal But out of Reach: Experiences from the National Network of Abortion Funds.* Hampshire, Mass., 1995.

North Dakota State Department of Health and Consolidated Laboratories. *Developmental Stages of Pregnancy.* Bismarck, N.D., 1992.

———. *Services Offered to Women and Children by Public and Private Agencies Statewide.* Bismarck, N.D., 1992.

Ohio Department of Health. *Fetal Development and Family Planning.* Columbus, Ohio, 1994.

———. *1995–96 Services Directory.* Columbus, Ohio, 1994.

Pennsylvania Department of Health. *Abortion: Making a Decision.* Harrisburg, Pa.

———. *Abortion: Making a Decision Directory of Services.* Harrisburg, Pa.

Petrillo, Lisa. "Selling Babies Is a Big Business for Bogus Abortion Clinics." *Ms.* September/October 1993.

Planned Parenthood of Houston and Southeast Texas. *First Trimester Abortion: A Patient Education Video.* Houston, Tex.

Reproductive Health Services. *Making A Choice.* St. Louis, Mo., 1994.

Routh Street Women's Clinic. *I Know I Made the Right Decision, But . . . Resolving Feelings about Abortion.* Dallas, Tex.

———. *Is There Love after Abortion?: Rebuilding Communication after a Difficult Decision.* Dallas, Tex.

———. *My Parents Would Kill Me: On Abortion, Especially for Teens.* Dallas, Tex.

Salo, Mark. *"Bogus" Abortion Referral Services and "Bogus" Clinics.* U.S. Congress. House Committee on Small Business. Subcommittee on Regulations, Business Opportunities and Energy, Washington, D.C.

Scoon-Rogers, Lydia, and Gordon H. Lester. *Child Support for Custodial Mothers and Fathers: 1991.* U.S. Department of Commerce, Washington, D.C., 1995.

South Carolina Department of Health and Environmental Control. *Directory of Services for Women, Children and Families.* Columbia, S.C., 1995.

———. *Embryonic and Fetal Development.* Columbia, S.C., 1995.

Tiamat, Uni M. *Herbal Abortion: The Fruit of the Tree of Knowledge.* Sage-femme! Peoria, Ill., 1994.

Utah Department of Health. *Information about the Developing Embryo and Fetus, about Abortion, and about Abortion Alternatives.* Salt Lake City, Utah, 1993.

Vaughan, Christopher. *How Life Begins: The Science of Life in the Womb.* Times Books, New York, 1996.

APPENDIX 3

SAMPLE FORMS

The forms in this appendix were developed by the National Abortion Federation and individual NAF members and are intended as samples only. The forms used by your provider may contain different wording and somewhat different information.

One-Parent Notification by Mail

Date: _____

Dear _____ ,

    Your daughter, _____ , has authorized me to advise you that she has made an appointment with our clinic for the purpose of terminating her pregnancy.

    Without your daughter's written consent, we are not able to discuss with you any specific information concerning her file. According to state law, we are required to notify a parent or legal guardian of a minor's intention to terminate her pregnancy. By law, parents of a minor child cannot withhold consent for the abortion. Once you have been notified, your daughter has the right to make her own decision.

Sincerely,

(Name of medical director) or (Name of director of facility)
Agent for (name of medical director)

Verification of Absent Parent's Signature
Certification of Written Notice

Patient's name: _____

    I certify that the attached written statement by my daughter's father/ mother (circle one), acknowledging her intent to terminate her pregnancy at *(insert name of clinic)* on _____ , was signed by him/her.

_____ Date _____

PARENT'S SIGNATURE

_____

ADDRESS AND PHONE

_____

_____

_____

WITNESS OR NOTARY PUBLIC

Two-Parent Consent in Clinic
(To be signed by both parents when accompanying a minor.)

We, _____ and _____ attest,

      (PRINT NAME OF MOTHER)   (PRINT NAME OF FATHER)

under penalty of perjury, that we are the lawful parents or legal guardians of _____ , and herewith give our consent for her to have an induced abortion. We understand that the doctor and facility providing the abortion procedure are relying on this statement to fulfill their legal obligations under *(insert state statute)*, and we agree to pay any expenses they incur as a result of this statement not being true.

_____   _____

SIGNATURE OF MOTHER   SIGNATURE OF FATHER

_____   _____

ADDRESS   ADDRESS

_____   _____

PHONE NUMBER   PHONE NUMBER

_____   _____

DATE   DATE

_____

WITNESS OR NOTARY PUBLIC

Two-Parent Notification in Clinic.
(To be signed by both parents accompanying a minor.)

Patient's name: _____

Parents' names: _____
                         MOTHER'S NAME

                         _____
                         ADDRESS

                         _____

                         _____
                         PHONE NUMBER

                         _____
                         FATHER'S NAME

                         _____
                         ADDRESS

                         _____

                         _____
                         PHONE NUMBER

The undersigned parents of _____ ,
                                        (DAUGHTER'S NAME)
age _____ , are aware of her pregnancy and her decision to have an abortion at the *(insert name of clinic)*. We understand that the doctor and facility providing the abortion procedure are relying on this statement to fulfill their legal obligations under *(insert state statute)*, and we agree to pay any expenses they incur as a result of this statement not being true.

_____ Date _____
MOTHER'S SIGNATURE

_____ Date _____
FATHER'S SIGNATURE

_____
WITNESS OR NOTARY PUBLIC

Sample Petition for Judicial Bypass

COUNTY COURT
JUVENILE DIVISION

In the Matter of the Petition of:

PETITION FOR PHYSICIAN'S
AUTHORIZATION

_____

Court File No. _____

To authorize physician to proceed with proposed abortion without prior parental notification.

PETITIONER'S NAME: _____

DATE OF BIRTH: _____

PETITIONER'S ADDRESS: _____

Petitioner moves the Court for authorization to her physician to be allowed to perform a proposed abortion upon said Petitioner without prior notification being required or given to Petitioner's parent(s), guardian, or custodian.

Petitioner bases her motion on one or more of the following alternative grounds:

1. That she is an emancipated minor;

2. That she is mature and capable of giving informed consent to the proposed abortion;

3. That it is within her best interest for the physician to perform the abortion upon Petitioner without prior notification of parent(s), guardian, or conservator.

Petitioner wishes to be represented in these proceedings by legal counsel, and does not have private counsel nor the funds with which to retain private counsel and therefore requests the Court to appoint legal counsel on her behalf.

THEREFORE, Petitioner requests an Order to authorize any physician associated with the Clinic to perform an abortion, including subsequent medical procedures required to assure that such pregnancy has been terminated upon her at her request and without prior notification being given to her parent(s), guardian, or conservator.

Noted this _____ day of _____ , 19 ___ .

_____

Petitioner

_____ , Petitioner, being first duly sworn on oath, states that she has read the foregoing petition subscribed by her, that she knows the contents thereof, and that the same is true to her best information and belief.

_____

Petitioner

Subscribed & sworn to before me

this _____ day of _____ , 19 ___ .

_____

Notary Public

Sample Medical Informed Consent Form

<u>ONE-DAY SURGERY</u>

<u>CONSENT TO OUTPATIENT VACUUM ASPIRATION (VA)</u>

<u>OR DILATION & EVACUATION (D&E) ONE-DAY ABORTION</u>   DATE _____

DO NOT SIGN THIS FORM WITHOUT READING AND UNDERSTANDING ITS CONTENTS

(OFFICE ONLY)–I.D. _____ VERIFICATION # _____

I, _____ , Age ____ , hereby give my consent to, and request and authorize
Dr. _____ and assistants of his/her choosing to perform an ABORTION on me.

<u>PATIENT</u>   <u>COUNSELOR</u>
Initial boxes   Initial boxes
as you read   as explained
                                                                           to patient

<u>DIAGNOSIS:</u> Tests and/or examinations have indicated that I am pregnant. I certify that the first day of my last normal menstrual period was (date) _____ .

<u>PURPOSE OF ABORTION:</u> I understand that the purpose of an abortion is to end my pregnancy.

<u>PROCEDURE:</u> It has been explained to me, and I understand, the operation consists of stretching open the mouth of the uterus (cervix), and with surgical instruments, removing the contents of my uterus. <u>LAMINARIA:</u> It has been explained to me that a local anesthesia may be administered and that one or more laminaria (which have been shown to me) may be inserted into the cervix in order to open it gently and slowly. I understand that once the laminaria are inserted, the abortion procedure has begun and therefore I MAY NOT CHANGE MY MIND. I will not leave the center until I am discharged by the medical staff. I understand that each laminaria has a string which may protrude from the vagina and that I am NOT to pull on the string(s). The laminaria absorbs moisture and enlarges the opening of the cervix and this may cause cramping, bleeding, or infection. The benefit of laminaria is to make the abortion procedure easier and reduce the possibility of other complications.

<u>REPEAT PROCEDURES:</u> I understand that it may become necessary to undergo more than one laminaria insertion. If so, I also understand that occasionally, subsequent re-insertions may have to be performed under general anesthesia and that these risks have been explained below under "Anesthesia Risks." I also understand that there may be an additional charge for this procedure.

<u>ALTERNATIVES:</u> I understand that the alternatives to abortion are either to have the baby and keep it, or have the baby and give it up for adoption. I have considered these alternatives and the staff here have offered to make referrals to appropriate agencies for birth and/or adoption. I reject these alternatives and request that the abortion procedure be performed.

<u>MATERIAL RISKS OF SURGERY:</u> As a result of surgical procedures, there may be material risks of: infection, allergic reaction, disfiguring scar, severe loss of blood, loss of or loss of function of limb or organ, paralysis, paraplegia or quadriplegia, brain damage, cardiac arrest, or death.

<u>ANESTHESIA RISKS:</u> I consent to the administration of anesthesia and authorize the use of such anesthetics as the doctor or anesthetist may decide, with the exception of: _____ . I understand that the risks of LOCAL anesthesia range from minor to severe, including but not limited to convulsions, cardiac arrest, and possibly the rare event of death. I understand the risks of GENERAL anesthesia range from minor (nausea, phlebitis) to severe (cardiac arrest, respiratory failure, prolonged unconsciousness), and even death. I warrant that I have not had anything at all to eat, no mints or gum, or drink since midnight last night with the exception of: _____ . I request (check one): GENERAL (asleep) anesthesia ( ) or LOCAL (awake) anesthesia ( ).

<u>RISKS OF ABORTION:</u> I understand that having an abortion involves risks to me, including but not limited to: hemorrhage, shock, cardiac arrest, uterine rupture,

Sample Medical Informed Consent Form, con't

sterility, amniotic fluid embolism, DIC (disseminated intravascular coagulation), or even death. Other risks: PERFORATION (puncture) of the uterus and/or bowel. In such event, hospitalization may be necessary for additional surgery. INFECTION: In order to avoid this complication, I agree to take the precautions explained to me and listed in the postoperative instructions entitled "How to Take Your Medications" and "What to Do After Your Procedure." INCOMPLETE ABORTION: In some instances, all tissue may not be removed and an incomplete abortion will result and the procedure may have to be repeated. I understand that there is no guarantee regarding the abortion and I may still be pregnant after the procedure or I may have fever, heavy bleeding, severe cramping, or pain. I agree that I will call the 24 hour emergency number given to me. MULTIPLE PREGNANCY: In the event of a multiple pregnancy, another abortion procedure may be required. ECTOPIC PREGNANCY: In some instances the pregnancy may occur in the fallopian tubes leading to the uterus and an abortion procedure cannot successfully terminate such a pregnancy, and that due to the threat of rupture to the tubes, immediate hospitalization may be necessary. I understand that the above complications might require a D&C or D&E procedure (cleaning out the uterus), a hysterectomy, or may result in permanent sterility or death. CERVICAL INCOMPETENCY: I understand that the abortion procedure (or repeated abortion procedures) may result in cervical incompetency which means that I may have problems maintaining a pregnancy in the future (possible miscarriage, stillbirth, low birth weight, premature delivery), or other complications in pregnancy. ASHERMAN'S SYNDROME: EMOTIONAL DISTRESS: I understand that depression or other emotional or psychological consequences may occur. I understand that I may call the 24 hour telephone number for follow-up counseling and referral. I ACCEPT ALL THESE RISKS.

PROGNOSIS: The likelihood of success of the above procedure is good ( ), fair ( ), poor ( ), provided aftercare instructions are followed and follow-up care is obtained. I understand that if I do not have the abortion procedure, the prognosis (predicted future medical condition) is continued pregnancy with the risks of same.

_____ M.D.

I understand that the practice of medicine is not an exact science and that NO GUARANTEES OR ASSURANCES HAVE BEEN MADE TO ME concerning the results of this procedure. I understand that the physician, medical personnel and other assistants will rely on statements I have made, the medical history I have given and other information in determining whether to perform the procedure or the course of treatment for me and I warrant that I have made full, complete and truthful disclosure.

ADDITIONAL PROCEDURES: If during the course of the abortion procedure, any unforseen conditions or complications arise, and the doctor in his/her professional medical judgment decides that different or additional procedures including but not limited to anesthesia or blood transfusion or the association of another doctor, or hospitalization at a hospital may be necessary, I give my consent to such. I assume all financial responsibility for payment for additional services. I give my permission for my parents (or legal guardian where applicable) or other person (name set forth below) to be notified by the doctor or staff member. The correct identity, address, and phone number of my emergency contact is set out below.

LABORATORY: I consent to diagnostic studies, tests, sonograms, x-ray examinations, and any other treatment or courses of treatment relating to the diagnosis of my condition or procedures set forth herein. I understand that the purpose of a sonogram here is to determine gestational size only and NOT to rule out or determine fetal abnormalities or deformities. I also consent to the disposal of any tissue or other parts of the contents of my uterus (womb) which may be removed during the abortion at the discretion of the physician or the clinic. I acknowledge that I may voluntarily receive tests for gonorrhea and syphilis and my doctor or his/her assistants or the staff of the clinic may provide necessary information to my State Department of Human Resources and I may be contacted for referral.

Sample Medical Informed Consent Form, con't

I also consent to the administration of RhoGam (or equivalent) should my blood be Rh negative. I agree that the doctor or clinic staff may need to contact me or my emergency contact regarding additional laboratory findings. My confidentiality will be respected where possible.

EMERGENCY: If I develop a fever, heavy bleeding, severe cramping, pain, or any other symptom, I agree to notify the clinic at once. I have been given an emergency telephone number which I can call 24 hours a day for assistance. My failure to give notice releases the doctor or clinic from any responsibility to me.

FOLLOW-UP: I have been advised to return to the clinic for a follow-up examination within 3 weeks after today. I understand that this exam is needed to be sure that no complications or other problems have appeared, that I am not still pregnant, and that the healing process has gone on properly. I agree to follow the instructions provided me and to take my medications as directed. I further agree to obtain the follow-up care either here or at some place else at my own expense. My failure to follow instructions or obtain care relieves the doctor and clinic of any responsibility to me.

I GIVE MY CONSENT FOR THE ABORTION FREELY AND WITHOUT COERCION.

By signing this form, I acknowledge that I have read or had this form explained to me, that I fully understand its contents, and that I have been given ample opportunity to ask questions and that any questions have been answered satisfactorily. All blanks or statements requiring completion were filled in and all statements I do not approve of were stricken before I signed this form. I also have received additional information including but not limited to the materials listed below relating to the procedure described herein. I understand that I can request and receive a sample copy of this consent if I choose to do so.

ADDITIONAL MATERIALS USED OR FURNISHED TO PATIENT:
What to Expect After the Procedure, How to Take Your Medications, Patient Feedback Sheet

_____

NOTIFY IN EMERGENCY OR IF PATIENT CANNOT BE REACHED	PATIENT'S SIGNATURE
Name _____	_____
Address _____	Address _____
City, State, Zip _____	City, State, Zip _____
Phone ( ) _____	Phone ( ) _____
Relationship _____	Counselor _____

ADULT'S CONSENT

I am the (relationship) _____ of the patient whose signature appears above. I have read and had explained to me the matters set forth in the above and hereby request and give my consent thereto and I agree to pay for all medical expenses incurred in this or as a result of this procedure.

PARENT'S, GUARDIAN'S, OR ADULT'S SIGNATURE

_____

Address _____

City, State, Zip _____

_____   Phone (   ) _____
Witness to Adult's Consent

_____

_____ M.D.

INDEX